# THE
# HEALTHY HEART
## HANDBOOK FOR
## WOMEN

*Life-saving strategies for
protection against heart disease*

# Dr David Ashton

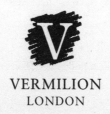

VERMILION
LONDON

1 3 5 7 9 10 8 6 4 2

Text © Dr David Ashton 2000

Dr David Ashton has asserted his right to be identified as the author of this work
under the Copyright, Designs and Patent Act 1988.

First published in 2000 by Vermilion
an imprint of Ebury Press
Random House, 20 Vauxhall Bridge Road, London SW1V 2SA

Random House Australia (Pty) Limited
20 Alfred Street, Milsons Point, Sydney, New South Wales 2061, Australia

Random House New Zealand Limited
18 Poland Road, Glenfield, Auckland 10, New Zealand

Random House South Africa (Pty) Limited
Endulini, 5A Jubilee Road, Parktown 2193, South Africa

The Random House Group Limited Reg. No. 954009

A CIP catalogue record for this book is available from the British Library.

ISBN 0 09 185610 8

Printed and bound in Great Britain by Mackays of Chatham plc, Kent

Papers used by Vermilion are natural, recyclable products made from wood
grown in sustainable forests.

*For Chrissie*

# Contents

# Acknowledgements

My interest in cardiovascular prevention started more than twenty five years ago when working as a junior hospital doctor in the cardiology department of a large teaching hospital. In those days, the science of prevention was in its infancy and my attempts to interest my colleagues in the subject were greeted with a mixture of apathy and amusement. Fortunately for me, even in those days there were several outstanding individuals who stimulated my interest and inspired me to continue working in this area. Professors Paul Durrington, Bruce Davies and, later, Professor David Wood, are all distinguished colleagues and friends who have contributed original work in the area of heart disease prevention and who have greatly influenced my own development.

My particular interest in heart disease in women started in the late 1980s, when I managed to convince the then Medical Director of Marks and Spencer, Dr Derek Taylor, that we should establish a major study into the causes of heart disease in women, with the Marks and Spencer female employees as the subjects. It was from that original study that the UK Women's Heart Study – based on more than 21,000 subjects – grew. I am, therefore, extremely grateful to Marks and Spencer for their generous support over many years and to the large numbers of women who have volunteered to participate in this important study.

It is in the nature of things that most of those involved in producing a book remain anonymous. There are, however, several individuals whose contribution has been exceptional and I am pleased to acknowledge them here.

As always Stephen Browne provided computer advice and solutions at all sorts of odd times, both day and night. Lyndell Costain, an independent consultant nutritionist, provided valuable comments on Part III of the mansucript and on several other sections covering nutritional issues. I am very grateful to them both.

Finally, I am indebted to my agent John Pawsey for his support and encouragement and also to my editor Joanna Carreras of Random House for her help, advice – and patience!

# Introduction

Whenever I ask a group of women what they believe to be the greatest threat to their long-term health, the chances are that cancer – and breast cancer, in particular – will be top of the list. So widespread is this perception that the truth often comes as something of a shock. For in reality a woman is *five times* more likely to die from heart disease than from breast cancer. Indeed, cardiovascular disease (heart attack and stroke) in women accounts for more deaths than *all* forms of cancer put together. So how is it possible that in this age of the Internet and global information exchange, women continue to exhibit such a worrying lack of awareness about this potentially life-threatening disease?

A significant part of the explanation lies in the way heart disease tends to be treated in the media. For the past two decades it has been portrayed almost exclusively as a male problem. Indeed, such has been the emphasis on heart disease in men that you could easily be forgiven for thinking that women rarely, if ever, become victims. After all, when did you last see a feature film or play, watch a TV soap or read a novel in which the heroine has a heart attack? Implicit in the message carried by TV and magazine articles is that it is a woman's responsibility to look after *his* heart. Health promotion initiatives have fared no better: they too have tended to emphasise heart disease in men and cancers in women.

Why have the media messages been so misleading? One explanation could be the fact that, until recently, most research studies into this subject have included only men – and middle-aged white men in particular. This could be because medicine has traditionally been a male-dominated profession, but the more likely explanation is that, on average, heart disease affects men ten years earlier than women. Thus, the social and economic consequences of premature illness and death due to heart disease in men have been greater than for women.

Whatever the reasons, the pervasive male bias in our perspective has important consequences. Because a woman tends to see cancer as a more significant health threat, she may be much less inclined to respond to health messages about heart disease if she does not see them as relevant to her. Importantly, she may be much less inclined to report symptoms of heart disease than her male counterpart. There is evidence to suggest that women take longer to reach hospital following a heart attack, perhaps because they have failed to recognise their symptoms as being heart-related. Furthermore, if doctors themselves receive similar male-orientated messages about heart disease, they too may disregard potentially serious symptoms in their female patients and be less inclined to offer preventive advice to them.

All this sounds pretty gloomy and it would be if there was nothing one could do about it. But now for the good news! The enormous amount of research into the causes of heart disease over the last fifty years has identified several key risk factors such as smoking, high blood cholesterol and raised blood pressure as powerful predictors of the disease in both men and women. In addition to these 'classical' risk factors affecting both sexes, there are additional factors, such as the menopause, hormone replacement therapy (HRT) and oral contraceptive history, which are specific to women, as well as others whose role is still under investigation. Because we now know a great deal about what causes heart disease in women, prevention and more effective treatment have become a reality. While a decade ago I would tell patients that *much* of the burden of heart disease was preventable, today I can say with confidence that *most* of it is, and even those who already have heart disease can look forward to a relatively normal life, thanks to modern drugs and surgery.

For these reasons, I believe a book on heart health specifically for women is timely. The very fact that you are reading this suggests that you have at least a passing interest in the subject, but if you already have some form of heart disease, then you have reason to pay more attention than most. And you are not alone. British women continue to have one of the highest rates of heart disease in the world and the lack of a co-ordinated effort to raise the level of awareness regarding the importance of cardiovascular disease in women, is clearly a serious and urgent public health issue.

At the time of writing, scientists from the Human Genome Project have announced that the first draft of the human genetic blueprint is complete. This is clearly an astonishing achievement and one that will provide unprecedented opportunities for even better prevention and treatment in the future. But, despite the achievements of medical science and technology, the health of human beings will ultimately always continue to depend primarily upon what we do – or don't do – for ourselves. Choices about diet, smoking and leisure-time physical activity will remain the strongest determinants of cardiovascular health for us all.

Whether you already have a heart condition and would like to reduce your risk of further problems, or whether you are simply interested in doing what you can to avoid heart disease altogether, my aim in this book is the same: *to provide the very best advice on how to reduce your risks of heart disease and to improve your overall quality of life.* Most of all, this is not a book about disease; the emphasis is very much on heart *health* and about informed choices. It is about what you *can do* for yourself, not the wishful, the fanciful or the unobtainable.

Dr David Ashton
November 2000

# PART I

# 1

# A woman's heart – anatomy of a disease

*My true love hath my heart, and I have his,*
*By just exchange one for another given*

Sir Philip Sidney (1554–86)

Since ancient times, the heart has occupied a central position in human beings' emotions, presumably because there is a readily apparent link between respiration, which depends upon the heart, and living. The vital part the heart plays in our individual and collective imaginations is illustrated by the extent to which we are still prepared to attribute to it all manner of mysteries and emotions, which do not have any basis in reality. Poets and songwriters have always talked about the lover's heart 'breaking' or 'aching', or even being left in San Francisco. Even today we still occasionally hear of someone dying of a 'broken heart'. The Greek physician Galen (AD 130–200) regarded the heart as a flame that heated the blood – an attitude, which, although less romantic, still has a certain appeal.

So what exactly *is* the human heart, this astonishing organ about which poets have been penning their immortal lines ever since language was invented? For astonishing it most certainly is.

## The normal heart

Every organ in the body needs a continuous supply of blood to function normally. Fresh blood brings oxygen and essential nutrients to the tissues, and takes away unwanted carbon dioxide and other waste products. This could not happen without the heart.

The heart is a muscular pump about the size of your fist and is situated in the middle of the chest, just to the left of centre (see Figure 1). It has four chambers, weighs around 10 oz and beats (on average) 70 times per minute, 100,000 times per day, or roughly 40 million times per year. During the average lifetime it will beat an awesome three billion times.

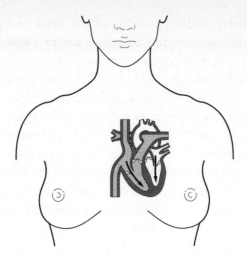

*Figure 1*  The position of the heart

The heart supplies oxygen-rich blood to every organ in the body, including itself, by pumping blood through the 96,000 km (60,000 miles) of blood vessels in the body. As a pumping mechanism it has a degree of efficiency which would amaze any engineer, and which is way beyond any man-made equivalent. It pumps about 7000 litres (1500 gallons) of blood every day. Given its amazing capacity, you might think that it would get its own supply of life-giving oxygen directly from the blood passing through it; but it doesn't. Instead, the heart muscle receives its own blood (and hence oxygen) supply via two small arteries that are about 3mm (1/8in) in diameter – the right and left coronary arteries (Figure 2).

*Figure 2*  The arterial blood supply to the heart

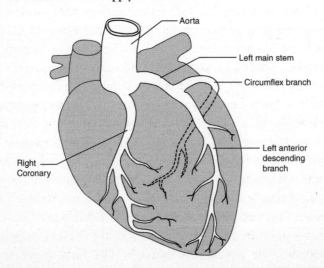

The two coronary arteries branch off the main blood vessel in the body, the aorta, and encircle the heart like a crown (the word coronary comes from the Latin word *corona*, meaning crown). The left coronary artery is the larger of the two, but divides soon after its origin into the left anterior descending and the left circumflex arteries. This is why doctors usually refer to three main coronary arteries, i.e. the right, the left anterior descending and the left circumflex. The right coronary artery supplies blood to the right side and back of the heart, while the two branches of the left coronary artery supply the front and left side of the heart. Because the heart relies so much on the coronary arteries for oxygen-rich blood, it is clearly vulnerable to any disease that may lead to damage or blocking of these arteries – and therein lies the problem.

# What is coronary heart disease?

Heart disease – or, more precisely, coronary heart disease (CHD) – is the name given to disease in one or more of the three coronary arteries referred to above. It is best understood as consisting of two key processes:

- The formation of plaque (fatty deposits) in the lining of the coronary artery.

- Rupture of the plaque and the subsequent development of a thrombosis (blood clot) in the artery.

### Plaque formation

In the newborn child, the inner lining of the coronary arteries is smooth, glistening and pearly white. The arteries themselves are flexible and supple and if they were to remain in this condition we would never have heard about heart disease or stroke. The problem is that because of our Western lifestyle, and diet in particular, the health of our arteries gradually deteriorates as we get older. For years the common metaphor for heart disease has been the clogged pipe: fat and cholesterol gradually accumulate in the wall of the artery reducing normal blood flow and, if a blood clot occurs, blocking the artery completely (see Figure 3). When this happens in the heart the result is a coronary thrombosis or heart attack (the medical term for which is myocardial infarction). The same process in blood vessels supplying the brain results in a stroke. Body tissues and organs deprived of oxygen can survive for a limited period only – a few minutes or so in the case of the brain. If the blood supply is not restored there will be permanent damage. The fatty deposits in the arteries are called plaque or, to use the correct medical term, atheroma, and the whole process is called atherosclerosis.

We now know that this is a simplified account of what actually happens. Although the degree of plaque formation is important in producing symptoms such as angina (chest pain) or shortness of breath, it is the *rupture* of unstable plaque (see below) that may actually precipitate an acute heart attack.

Several other points about plaque formation are important:

- The more plaque there is, the greater the risk of heart attack, stroke or symptoms such as angina.
- Individuals who have known coronary risk factors such as cigarette smoking, high blood pressure or diabetes have more plaque than those who do not.
- Because a woman's heart is smaller and has narrower coronary arteries than a man's, it takes less plaque to block them.

## Plaque rupture and thrombosis

It is now clear that the rupture of plaque that has become unstable causes 60–70 per cent of heart attacks. Moreover, even plaque which is not large enough to impede blood flow to the heart in its own right can rupture and lead to thrombosis and complete blockage of an artery.

Plaque formation and thrombosis are closely linked. During the first thirty or forty years of our lives, most of us are accumulating varying amounts of plaque in our arteries. Once this has become established, the stage is set and we are then highly vulnerable to factors that can cause plaque instability and rupture. When the plaque breaks, it releases several complex chemical messengers, which trigger a cascade of events leading to thrombosis and complete blockage of the artery (see Figure 3).

*Figure 3*  **Plaque formation, rupture and thrombosis in a coronary artery**
In childhood, the endothelium (lining of the artery) is smooth and the artery is flexible (a). With advancing age and risk factors, fatty deposits and cells accumulate in the arterial wall – this is called plaque or atheroma (b). At this stage, symptoms of heart disease such as angina may become evident. As the process continues, areas of plaque may become unstable and rupture (c), leading to the formation of thrombosis (blood clot) and blockage of the artery (d). This is called a heart attack, coronary thrombosis or myocardial infarction.

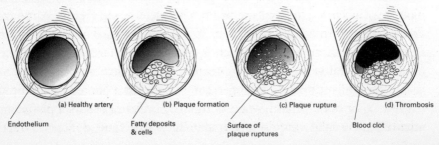

(a) Healthy artery          (b) Plaque formation          (c) Plaque rupture          (d) Thrombosis

Endothelium          Fatty deposits & cells          Surface of plaque ruptures          Blood clot

# What are the symptoms?

The three most important manifestations of CHD are angina (chest pain), unstable angina and heart attack.

## Angina

When blood flow to the heart is restricted due to plaque formation in the coronary arteries, angina may be the result. This normally means that one or more of the coronary arteries has a severe degree of blockage – more than 75 per cent of its normal diameter. The pain arises from the muscle fibres of the heart which have insufficient oxygen for the work they do. The harder the heart muscle works, the more oxygen will be required and the greater the imbalance between oxygen supply and demand. This is why angina is typically related to exertion such as walking up a hill or stairs, or carrying shopping, etc. It may also be precipitated by anxiety and stress. Angina pain usually subsides after a few minutes' rest. It is often worse in cold weather and if you exercise after a meal.

The pain itself is typically described as a crushing or gripping pain, or a feeling as though a tight band has been put across the chest (the word angina comes from the Latin *angere*, which means to strangle). Sometimes there is a sensation of 'pins and needles' in the left arm, or both arms. The chest discomfort may also radiate into the teeth or throat and be accompanied by breathlessness and sweating.

However, while these are the classical symptoms of angina in both sexes, it is important to recognise that women often have fewer typical symptoms of cardiac disease. Women with angina may complain of heaviness between the breasts, a 'sinking feeling', and weakness or a burning sensation rather than the constricting pain that men often report. In addition, breathlessness, mid-back pain, fatigue, indigestion and palpitations in women can also sometimes be signs of heart trouble, although in most cases such symptoms are entirely benign.

There is another type of chest pain known as Syndrome X or variant angina, which is more common in women. Syndrome X mimics cardiac pain, but when a coronary angiogram (special X-ray of the coronary arteries) is performed, the arteries are found to be normal. In some studies up to 40 per cent of women investigated for chest pain turn out to have perfectly normal coronary arteries (compared with only eight per cent of men). The cause of Syndrome X is not entirely clear, hence the name, but it is thought to be due to spasm in the coronary arteries rather than plaque or atheroma. It usually runs a benign course but is sometimes difficult to treat.

## Unstable angina

Angina is usually a fairly predictable symptom, but when the arterial narrowing is severe, the disease can enter a new phase – unstable angina. Unlike normal angina, the pain of unstable angina may occur after only minimal exertion or even at rest. It can also sometimes occur in bed at night, causing disturbed sleep patterns. Unstable angina can lead to a heart attack and preventive action is urgently required.

## The heart attack

When the degree of narrowing of the coronary arteries is severe, or if there has been rupture of plaque, a thrombosis (blood clot) may form and block the artery. This is a heart attack or myocardial infarction. Heart attacks can strike anywhere, day or night, at rest or during exercise. One minute the heart may be working perfectly normally, the next a blood clot has formed and the heart muscle is under serious threat. Symptoms may be dramatic, involving a sudden onset of excruciating chest pain accompanied by sweating and acute breathlessness. However, in many cases it may feel like little more than a prolonged attack of angina, and in some it may even be completely silent. Up to 35 per cent of heart attacks in women go unreported. Because of the considerable variation in severity of symptoms, diagnosis may be extremely difficult, even for an experienced doctor. *It is important to remember that a heart attack may occur*

*Figure 4*   **The heart attack (myocardial infarction)**
In (a) a relatively small artery has become blocked and a small area of the heart muscle has been lost. In (b) a larger vessel is involved and there is extensive loss of myocardium. A lesion at (c) implicates most of the heart and is potentially lethal.

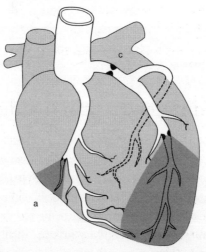

*without warning and in the absence of any previous symptoms of heart disease such as angina or breathlessness.*

The outcome for any woman suffering a heart attack will depend on both the site and the size of the artery involved (see Figure 4). Clearly, a complete blockage of the left coronary artery before its division would threaten the whole of the left side of the heart and could be fatal. Conversely, a small clot in a small branch of the right coronary artery is unlikely to cause much damage, allowing a full recovery in most cases.

One of the most significant advances in the modern treatment of the acute heart attack has been the advent of 'clot busting' drugs called thrombolytics, which, if given within the first few hours, can stop a heart attack in its tracks by dissolving the clot. The use of these drugs has reduced the heart attack death rate by 20 per cent. The main warning symptoms of a heart attack are summarised in the table below.

*Table 1*  **Warning symptoms of a heart attack in women**

*Common symptoms*
- uncomfortable pressure, fullness, crushing sensation or severe pain in the centre of the chest that lasts for more than a few minutes, or goes away and comes back
- pain spreading to shoulders, neck, arms or jaw with 'pins and needles'
- chest discomfort with light headedness, fainting, sweating, nausea, or shortness of breath

*Other symptoms*
- vague chest, stomach or abdominal pain
- nausea or dizziness
- shortness of breath and difficulty breathing
- unexplained anxiety, weakness or fatigue
- palpitations, cold sweat or pallor

*Note:* Not all of these symptoms occur in every attack. Sometimes they may go away and return. If symptoms persist consult your doctor.

# Gender differences in heart disease

It is now clear that there are important differences between the sexes in terms of symptoms, treatment and outcomes for coronary disease. For example, although women have a lower risk of dying from CHD than men for any given age, this survival advantage is lost once a woman develops symptoms of disease.

The most important gender differences with regard to CHD are summarised in Table 2 overleaf.

*Table 2*   Coronary heart disease – women vs. men

*Anatomy*
- Women have smaller hearts and narrower coronary arteries than men; hence less plaque is needed to produce blockage

*Symptoms*
- Women with angina may not have the classic symptoms of chest, arm or jaw pain. They may instead have less usual symptoms such as shortness of breath, fatigue, abdominal or back pain
- Angina is more likely to be the initial manifestation of CHD in women than men, whereas a heart attack is a more common first manifestation of heart disease in a man
- Syndrome X (anginal pain in the presence of normal coronary arteries) is much more common in women than men
- Women with heart disease may feel more chest pain during mental stress than men
- Women have a higher rate of unrecognised heart attack than men

*Diagnosis*
- Women with symptoms may be less likely than men to be referred for specialist assessment and diagnostic procedures

*Treatment*
- Women may be less likely to receive modern 'clot busting' drugs and surgical procedures designed to improve blood flow to the heart

*Outcomes*
- A woman is twice as likely as a man to die from a first heart attack
- A woman has a much greater risk of a second heart attack than a man
- Before 50, sudden death from a heart attack is four times more common in men than women
- Women with symptoms of chronic heart failure live twice as long as their male counterparts
- Women now do just as well as men after undergoing surgical procedures to restore normal blood flow to the heart e.g. coronary bypass and angioplasty

Some of these differences can be explained in terms of the quality of medical care provided. For example, until quite recently, almost all studies showed that women undergoing heart surgery had an in-hospital death-rate two-and-a-half times higher than that of men. Today, thanks to advances in technology, improved surgical techniques and possibly doctors' greater sensitivity to gender differences in heart disease, women now seem to do just as well as men after surgical procedures such as coronary bypass and angioplasty (see pp. 59–60) which help restore normal blood flow to the heart. Lower rates of referral for specialist assessment may simply reflect a lack of awareness among many doctors of the importance of coronary heart disease in women.

However, other gender variations point to real differences in the underlying disease process, some of which may be attributable to female-specific risk factors such as the menopause and hormone replacement therapy. In addition, women may respond differently to many of the powerful drugs used to treat the various symptoms of heart disease, such as angina and disturbances in the normal rhythm of the heart.

Whatever the complex factors involved, these gender differences are currently the subject of intense research in major centres all over the world. In the near future, a deeper understanding of the underlying disease processes in women will begin to make gender-specific prevention and treatment a reality. In the meantime, however, there is an enormous amount to be done in terms of heart disease prevention in women – the subject of the second part of this book.

# 2

# Vital statistics

*He uses statistics as a drunken man uses lampposts –*
*for support rather than illumination.*

Anon.

Not everyone finds statistics interesting but, for those who do, here are some of the latest facts and figures about coronary heart disease (CHD) and stroke in women*. Firstly, a brief word about terminology.

The term 'cardiovascular disease' (CVD) is a collective one which includes coronary heart disease (CHD), stroke and all other diseases of the heart and circulation, such as birth defects, rheumatic heart disease etc (see Figure 5). CHD and stroke are the two most common forms of CVD; between them they account for about three quarters of all CVD deaths. In this brief review, figures for all CVD will be given first, followed by the specific data for CHD and stroke. Morbidity means the number of people in the community with heart or circulatory disease. The term includes survivors of a heart attack or stroke and also those with angina, high blood pressure, arterial disease of the legs and heart failure. Mortality refers to the number of *deaths* from heart or circulatory diseases.

*Figure 5*

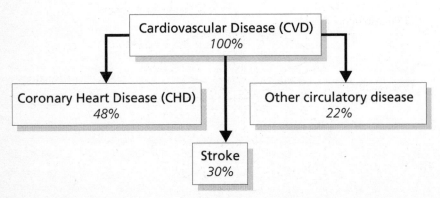

*NB. Primary sources: British Heart Foundation Statistics database 1999 and American Heart Foundation Statistics 2000.

# Cardiovascular disease (CVD)

- CVD is the main cause of death among women and men in the UK. In 1997, CVD accounted for over 260,000 deaths, more than half of which (52 per cent) were in women.
- Each day, approximately 375 women die from CVD in the UK – and that's one death every four minutes.
- CVD death rates in women lag behind those of men at all ages, even in the oldest age group (see Figure 6).

*Figure 6*   CVD death rates (per 100) by age for men and women

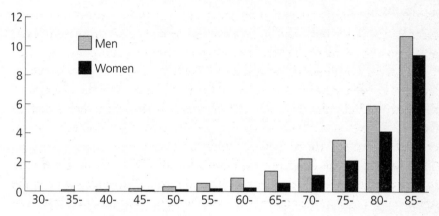

- Deaths due to CVD amounted to around 42 per cent of all causes of death in women – almost twice as many as were due to all forms of cancer (see Figure 7).

*Figure 7*   Major causes of death in UK women 1997

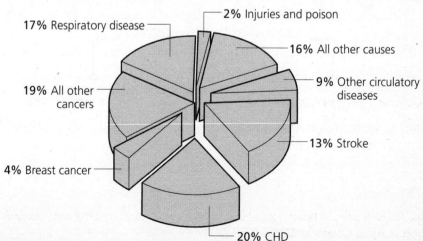

- CVD is the main cause of premature death (before age 75) in the UK; 30 per cent of premature deaths in women are from CVD.
- Including self-reported high blood pressure, 28 per cent of women in the UK report having been diagnosed with some form of CVD.
- According to the most recent calculations, if all major forms of CVD were eliminated, life expectancy would rise by almost seven years. If all forms of cancer were eliminated, the gain would be three years.

# Coronary heart disease (CHD)

### 1. Deaths in the UK
- CHD is, by itself, the commonest cause of death in the UK. In 1997, 64,000 women died from CHD.
- One in five women and one in four men will die from the disease.
- CHD is the most common cause of premature death (before age 75) in the UK; 17 per cent of premature deaths in women are from CHD.
- In two thirds (63 per cent) of women who die suddenly from CHD there were no previous symptoms of disease.

### 2. Deaths by age and sex
- Almost 75 per cent of all CHD deaths in women occur in those aged 75 years and over, compared with 50 per cent of deaths in men.
- Seven per cent of deaths due to CHD in women occur under the age of 65 years, compared with 20 per cent of deaths in men.
- Because CHD occurs later in women, the risk of death is roughly similar to that of men 10 years younger.

### 3. Following a heart attack
- Immediate mortality due to a heart attack is twice as high in women as in men.
- Women have a greater risk than men of suffering a further attack.
- Within six years after a recognised heart attack:
    33 per cent of women will have another attack
    15 per cent will develop angina
    13 per cent will have a stroke
    30 per cent will be disabled with cardiac failure
    Seven per cent will experience sudden cardiac death

### 4. Morbidity
- Approximately five per cent of women in the UK aged 25 years and over have suffered a heart attack or have angina.

- Between 1981/1982 and 1991/1992 there was a 31 per cent reduction in the reported number of women experiencing a heart attack, but a 69 per cent increase in the number of women having angina.

## 5. UK trends

- Death rates for CHD have been falling in the UK since the late 1970s (see Figure 8). Part of this improvement is due to the advent of better medical treatment, including new drugs.

*Figure 8*   Death rates from CHD, women aged 35–74, 1968–1994, UK*

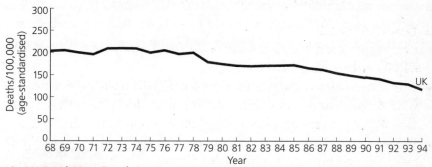

*Source:* British Heart Foundation

- Although the number of deaths due to CHD in women is falling, morbidity – due to angina, heart failure and other problems – is increasing (see morbidity opposite).

## 6. CHD vs. cancer

- CHD kills *three times* more women than cancer of the breast, ovary, and cervix combined.
- A woman is nearly five times more likely to die from CHD than from breast cancer.

## 7. CHD and social class

- There is a strong social class gradient for CHD deaths in women. For premature death, women in unskilled, manual occupations have twice the death rate of those in skilled, non-manual occupations.
- Women working in manual occupations report rates of morbidity from CHD and other diseases of the circulatory system which are 30 per cent higher than those in skilled, non-manual occupations.

## 8. Regional differences

- The highest death rates from CHD are found in Scotland, followed by Northern England and Northern Ireland. The lowest rates are found in the South of England and East Anglia.

- The premature death rate for women living in the north of England is almost 90 per cent higher than for women in East Anglia.

### 9. Ethnic differences

- South Asian women living in the UK (Indians, Bangladeshis, Pakistanis and Sri Lankans) have a 50 per cent higher premature death rate than average.
- Women from West Africa and the Caribbean have CHD rates which are significantly lower than average.

### 10. International comparisons

- Despite recent improvements, the death rate from CHD in the UK is still among the highest in the world (see Figure 9). It is exceeded only by some of the countries in Eastern and Central Europe, where deaths have been rising rapidly.

*Figure 9*   Death rates from CHD, men and women aged 35–74, 1993, selected countries*

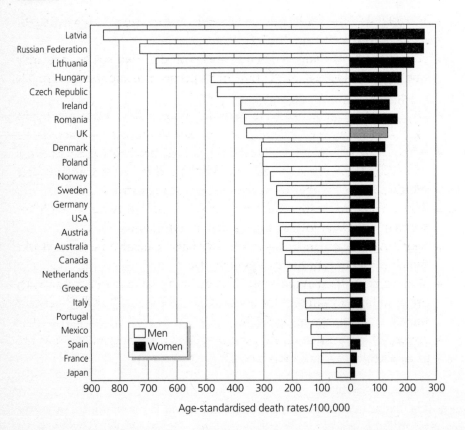

*Source:* British Heart Foundation

- Although the death rate from CHD has been falling in the UK, this fall has not been as fast as that in some other countries. Between 1984 and 1994, the death rate in women fell by 29 per cent in the UK but in Australia, France and Canada the rate fell by 45, 41 and 38 per cent respectively.

**11.  Economic consequences**
- CHD has major economic consequences for the UK as well as human costs.
- Costs to the healthcare system in the UK in 1996 were £1.6 billion.
- Production losses from death and illness due to CHD in 1996 cost the UK economy £8.5 billion.
- In summary, CHD is estimated to cost the UK economy in excess of £10 billion a year.

# Stroke

- In 1997, 41,000 deaths in women were due to stroke – accounting for around 30 per cent of all CVD deaths.
- Almost twice as many women as men will die from stroke, probably due to their older age at the time of its occurrence and their longer life expectancy.
- Death rates from stroke have been declining in both sexes; for adults aged 16–64 they have fallen by 28 per cent in the last 10 years.
- Although death rates from stroke are falling, morbidity from stroke is increasing. Between 1981/82 and 1991/92 there was a 50 per cent increase in the number of women experiencing a stroke.
- The premature death rate from stroke is nearly twice as high for women in manual jobs as for women in non-manual jobs.
- South Asian women living in the UK have a death rate from stroke which is 40 per cent higher than average.
- Women from West Africa and the Caribbean have stroke rates which are even higher than that for South Asian women – 80 and 57 per cent higher than average respectively.
- About 70 per cent of stroke victims survive the event, and women are more likely to survive than men.

# 3

# Heart disease – risks and reasons

In 1948, a small American town called Framingham, situated about 18 miles west of Boston, Massachusetts, was chosen as the location for a major study into the causes of heart disease and stroke. Some 5000 Framingham residents (2873 women and 2336 men) were recruited into the project and then followed up for symptoms of cardiovascular disease (angina, heart attack and stroke) over several decades. By comparing those who developed disease with those who did not, researchers were able to identify several risk factors associated with an increased risk of CVD, among them cigarette smoking, high blood cholesterol and raised blood pressure. It was, in fact, the Framingham researchers who, in 1961, first proposed the term 'risk factor', which is now so widely used by health professionals and lay people alike. Remarkably, the Framingham Heart Study continues to this day and, while scores of other studies from all over the world have since added to our understanding of the causes of heart disease, it is Framingham that remains the most important source of our knowledge about risk factors. It is also a tribute to the founders of the project that they were the first major study to include women in the study group; had they not done so, our knowledge concerning female-specific risk factors would be far less reliable than it is today.

This chapter provides a brief overview of the most important risk factors in women and their relationship with CVD, including some which have only recently been identified. Where appropriate, practical strategies to modify these factors are discussed in more detail in Part II of the book, under the relevant Action Files. For the purposes of the present discussion, risk factors can be divided into two main groups: modifiable and non-modifiable.

## Non-modifiable risk factors

Non-modifiable factors, as their name implies, are those, which while being important predictors of heart disease, cannot be altered by lifestyle changes or medical treatment. They are as follows:

## Age

Sadly, the arrow of time travels in only one direction – at least in our bit of the universe. We all grow older and, in the process, the risk of disease increases. Age is the strongest predictor of coronary deaths in women; more than four out of five women who die from heart disease are aged 65 years or older.

## Gender

There is no doubt that being male is a big disadvantage in the heart attack stakes. Before the age of 65, death rates in men are three to five times higher than those in women. Thus heart disease tends to affect men at the most economically productive time in their lives. Nevertheless, more than 4000 women a year will die from heart disease before they reach 65 and one quarter of these will be women under 55.

## Family history

As with age and gender, we didn't choose our parents and so we are stuck with our genetic history. If your mother or sister developed heart disease before 65, or your father or brother before 55, then your own risk of heart problems is significantly increased. A history of heart trouble in a second degree (grandparent, aunt, uncle) or third degree relative (cousin), is much less important. Having heart disease in the family may sound like bad news, but do remember that this does not mean you *will* develop similar problems, only that your risk of so doing is higher than average. In fact, most of the factors which increase the risk of heart disease are not genetic in origin and can be modified by relatively modest changes in lifestyle and, where required, modern drug therapy.

## Polycystic Ovarian Syndrome (PCOS)

Polycystic Ovarian Syndrome, or PCOS, is a common condition affecting five to ten per cent of women of child-bearing age. It causes the following symptoms:

- obesity
- acne and/or hirsutism (excessive body hair)
- infertility
- absent or abnormal periods
- enlarged ovaries with multiple cysts found on ultrasound examination.

PCOS is probably caused by genetic factors and often becomes evident around puberty. The reason why this is important to our discussion of CHD risk factors, is because a characteristic feature of PCOS is insulin resistance (see p.39). We know that individuals with raised insulin levels have a greatly increased CHD risk due to abnormal blood lipids (low HDL-C and raised triglycerides), hypertension (raised blood pressure) and an increased clotting tendency. These changes translate into a significantly increased risk of CHD in women with PCOS, possibly by as much as seven times greater than women without the condition. Effective management of PCOS requires advice from a physician with a special interest in this condition. (See Appendix 1, p.232, for The PCOS/Self-Help Group.)

# Modifiable risk factors

Modifiable risk factors are those that can be influenced by changes in various lifestyle-related behaviours, such as diet and exercise, and by medical treatment. Modifiable factors can be divided into two further groups: *major* and *contributory*.

## MAJOR MODIFIABLE RISK FACTORS

Major modifiable risk factors are those where the scientific evidence is very strong and where the contribution to risk is large. The main ones are as follows:

### Cigarette smoking

Cigarette smoking remains the leading preventable cause of CHD in women, with more than 50 per cent of heart attacks in middle-aged women attributable to tobacco. Although smoking was widespread among men at the turn of the last century, it was not until the 1920s that it became socially acceptable, indeed fashionable, among women. By the 1950s and 1960s, smoking had reached a peak with around 40 per cent of women being regular smokers.

Until recently the proportion of adult cigarette smokers had been declining, but at the time of writing it has levelled off. In 1996, 28 per cent of women and 29 per cent of men still smoked cigarettes (see Figure 10 opposite), although it should be noted that the smoking rates vary according to social class, with women in unskilled occupations smoking more than those in professional groups.

*Figure 10*  Cigarette smoking among adults aged 16 and over, 1972–1996, England*

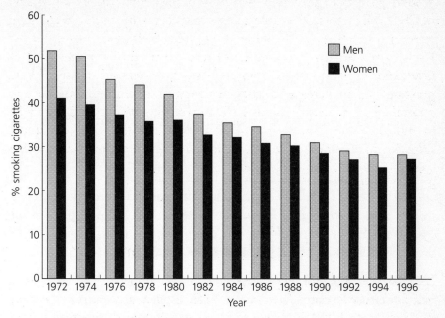

*Sources:* Data from Office for National Statistics (General Household Survey); analysis by Central Health Monitoring Unit, Department of Health.

Of concern is the fact that teenagers, particularly girls, are smoking more. In 1988, nine per cent of girls in England were regular smokers, but by 1996 this had risen to 15 per cent – an increase of 60 per cent. Among 16–19-year-old women in Great Britain, 28 per cent were regular smokers in 1988, rising to 32 per cent in 1996.

The number of cigarettes smoked is reflected in the risks. The more you smoke, the greater the risk of angina and heart attack (both fatal and non-fatal). Even smoking fewer than five cigarettes a day more than doubles the risk of heart disease. For women smoking 35 or more cigarettes per day, there is a seven-fold increase in risk for CHD. Diabetic women who also smoke seem particularly vulnerable to heart disease.

Overall, smoking triples the risk for heart attack, even among pre-menopausal women. It is also an important contributor to sudden cardiac death in young women. Cardiovascular risk is increased in women who both smoke and use oral contraceptives. There is, incidentally, no evidence to suggest that smoking cigarettes with reduced nicotine or tar levels lowers the coronary risk of smoking. (See Action File 1, p.93, on how to stop smoking.)

## Hypertension (raised blood pressure)

Blood pressure simply refers to the force of blood pushing against the walls of the arteries. It is measured in millimetres of mercury (or mm Hg) and the readings are written as two numbers, e.g. 122/78 mm Hg, both of which are important to your health. The top number is the systolic blood pressure (SBP), which is the pressure in the arterial system when the heart beats (contracts). The bottom number is the diastolic blood pressure (DBP), which is the pressure in the arteries when the heart rests between beats.

Hypertension – the medical term for high blood pressure – can be defined in different ways, depending upon which cut-offs are chosen for normal SBP and DBP. The current guidelines define normal blood pressure as up to 139/89 mm Hg and hypertension as a blood pressure of 140/90 mmHg or above. Using this definition, the latest survey (1998) shows that one-third of women aged 16 years and over, are hypertensive.

### Hypertension, age and social class

Blood pressure levels rise with age and, as a consequence, the proportion of individuals with hypertension also increases. In the latest survey, 78 per cent of women aged 75 years and over were classified as hypertensive, compared with only four per cent aged 16-24 years. The proportion of women with hypertension tends to be lower than that in men until around the age of 50, when the difference becomes less marked (see Figure 11).

As with cigarette smoking, there is a strong social class gradient, with hypertension being much more common in manual and unskilled occupations, compared with women in professional and managerial groups.

*Figure 11*  **Proportion of females and males with high blood pressure**

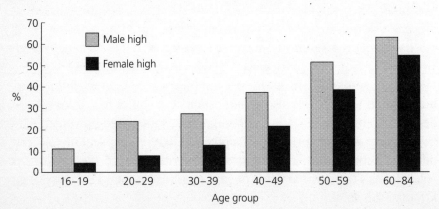

## Hypertension and CVD

Hypertension appears to accelerate the development of arterial plaque and places an additional strain on the heart, which has to pump against a much greater pressure in the arterial system. Because of this, hypertension is strongly associated with coronary heart disease and is *the* most important risk factor for stroke and heart failure. A rise of 10 mm Hg in SBP and/or DBP increases the risk of CVD in women by 20–30 per cent. In general, SBP appears to be a better predictor of risk in women than DBP. There is also a form of high blood pressure known as 'isolated systolic hypertension' (ISH) which occurs when the systolic pressure is high, but the diastolic pressure is normal. This, too, increases the risk of heart attack and stroke. Studies show that ISH affects 30 per cent of women over 65.

Hypertension is, therefore, a major cause of preventable disease. Of the one-third of women in this country who are hypertensive, many are receiving either inadequate treatment or no treatment at all. (See Action File 3, p.118, for information on how to achieve and maintain a healthy blood pressure.)

# Raised blood cholesterol

You may have heard the term 'blood lipids', which is the medical name given to all the fatty substances in the blood, including blood cholesterol. The various blood lipids have a crucial part to play in the development of heart disease and are discussed in detail in Action File 2.

For the purposes of the present discussion, the main lipid measurements to consider are as follows:

- *Blood cholesterol*: refers to the total amount of cholesterol in the blood (i.e. the sum of LDL-cholesterol, HDL-cholesterol and the small amounts contained in other blood lipids). Hence blood cholesterol is usually referred to as 'total cholesterol' (TC).
- *Low-density lipoprotein cholesterol* (LDL-C): the main form of cholesterol in the blood, high levels of which are associated with an increased risk of heart attack. For this reason it is also called 'bad cholesterol'.
- *High-density lipoprotein cholesterol* (HDL-C): often called the 'good cholesterol' since, unlike LDL-C, high levels actually protect against heart disease.
- *Triglycerides*: another form of blood lipid, high levels of which appear to increase the risk of heart disease in women, but not in men.

Blood cholesterol levels – TC, LDL-C and HDL-C – and triglycerides are measured by a blood test and the results are expressed in millimoles per litre (mmol/L). The ideal total cholesterol level for the population is less than 5.0 mmol/L. Currently, well over half the women in the UK have levels above this and the average value for women is 5.6 mmol/L.

### Cholesterol and age

Both TC and LDL-C levels rise gradually with age in women until they reach 50, after which a steeper increase is seen (see Figure 12a below). In fact, before the age of 50 men have higher cholesterol levels than women, whereas from 50 onwards, women have higher levels than men. This may help to explain why heart attack deaths among women rise so steeply in the sixth decade of life.

*Figure 12a*   Cholesterol levels by age*

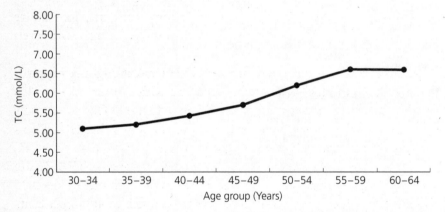

*Figure 12b*   HDL-C levels by age*

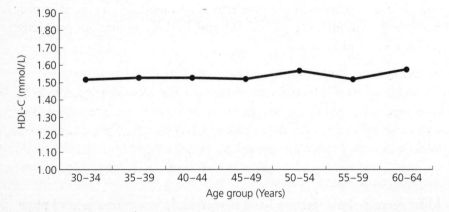

*Sources:* UK Women's Heart Study

Although it is often stated that HDL-C levels fall after the menopause, this is not the case. In fact, unlike TC and LDL-C, HDL-C levels are much more stable throughout life (see Figure 12b). Moreover levels of HDL-C in women are consistently higher than in men, which may also contribute to the lower rates of heart disease in women before middle age.

## Cholesterol and CHD risk

There is abundant evidence to show that the risk of CHD rises as total cholesterol (TC) and LDL-C levels increase. For example, in the Framingham Heart study, women with a TC level above 6.8 mmol/L had a heart attack risk two to three times higher than women with levels below 5.3 mmol/L. However, the increase in CHD risk observed for both TC and LDL-C is much smaller in women aged 65 and above, than in younger women. It is also important to note that at any given cholesterol level, the risk for a woman is significantly lower than that for a man. In the Framingham study, women with cholesterol concentrations above 7.6 mmol/L had heart attack rates lower than those for men with levels less than 5.3 mmol/L.

Because HDL-C is the 'good' form of cholesterol, it might be expected that high levels of HDL-C would be associated with a *lower* risk of CHD, i.e. the reverse of the position with TC and LDL-C. This is precisely what the evidence shows. Many studies have confirmed that HDL-C is a particularly powerful CHD risk factor in women – more than either TC or LDL-C. This means that even quite modest changes in HDL-C can have a very large impact on CHD risk. For example, a change of just 0.25 mmol/L can reduce or increase CHD risk by as much as 40-50 per cent.

Furthermore, high levels of HDL-C are protective even in women with raised TC levels. In other words, high blood levels of HDL-C appear to neutralise the potentially adverse effects of raised TC levels. It is also interesting that HDL-C, unlike TC and LDL-C, retains its predictive power even in older women.

## Triglycerides

The other form of blood fat to consider is the blood triglyceride level. Although not a significant risk factor in men, raised triglyceride levels in women do appear to increase the risk of CHD independently of other risk factors, in some studies by as much as 40 per cent.

## Physical inactivity

Most surveys show that we have a worryingly low proportion of physically active adults in this country, with the majority of the population

*Figure 13*  Proportion of women and men taking aerobic exercise
(5+ occasions/week)*

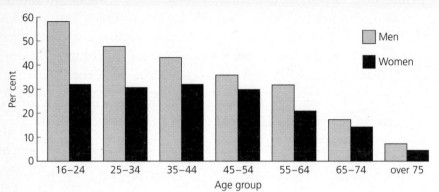

*Source:* Health Survey for England, 1998.

failing to take even the minimum amount of exercise needed to achieve a
health benefit. Only around 20 per cent of women in the UK are active
enough to give themselves some protection against CHD. Not that we're
alone; similar surveys in Canada, Australia and the USA indicate that a
sedentary lifestyle travels well, since the levels of physical activity (or
inactivity) are broadly the same as in the UK.

Participation in aerobic activity declines with age. Participation rates,
however, are lower in women than men at any given age (see Figure 13).
Most vigorous exercise is achieved through sport and exercise during
leisure time but, despite a widespread perception to the contrary, the
number of women participating in sports, games or other physical activities is not increasing significantly. There is also a social class difference in
activity patterns, with participation rates considerably higher among
women in professional or skilled occupations than among those engaged
in manual or unskilled work.

Partly as a consequence of low activity levels, fitness levels are also low.
It is estimated that two-thirds of women cannot sustain a normal walking pace up a gradual slope (i.e. a five per cent gradient at three mph)
without becoming breathless and having to stop to avoid discomfort.

### Physical activity and CHD risk

Although there are fewer studies on the relationship between physical
activity and heart disease in women compared with men, the conclusions
are broadly the same: women who are physically active have a 50 per cent
reduction in coronary risk compared with their inactive counterparts.
Even in older women, a decrease of about 50 per cent in heart attack

risk results from modest, habitual leisure-time activities, such as 30–45 minutes of brisk walking three times weekly.

## Diabetes

In normal circumstances, the body monitors the amount of sugar in the blood. After eating, levels of blood sugar in the body rise. When this happens, the pancreas releases insulin into the bloodstream. Insulin is a hormone that helps to remove sugar from the bloodstream into the body's cells, a crucial part of the fine balancing act that regulates the use of energy. If insulin is either deficient or ineffective, blood sugar levels rise, sugar (glucose) appears in the urine and the signs and symptoms of diabetes appear. There are two main types of diabetes: Type I and Type II.

Type I – insulin-dependent diabetes or 'juvenile onset' diabetes – usually begins in childhood or early adulthood and has a strong genetic component. This form of diabetes is due to destruction of the cells in the pancreas and is characterised by a complete lack of insulin, which must, therefore, be supplied by regular injections.

Type II – non-insulin dependent diabetes (NIDDM), or 'maturity-onset' diabetes – tends to develop in middle-aged or older individuals, particularly those who are obese (see p.38). In this type of diabetes the pancreas still secretes adequate amounts of insulin, but because the cells seem resistant to its effects, the body tries to overcome the resistance by releasing even more insulin into the bloodstream. Thus, in contrast to individuals with Type I diabetes, where insulin levels are low or absent, those with Type II diabetes often have higher than normal blood insulin levels. Most cases of Type II diabetes can be managed with a combination of diet, exercise and oral medication (hence the term non-insulin dependent). In practice, a small proportion may also require insulin.

In the UK, approximately 1.4 million people have diabetes and this figure is set to more than double in the next decade. About 95 per cent of cases are Type II or non-insulin dependent diabetes. The reason why diabetes is such an important condition is because it greatly increases the risk of CVD – including heart attack, stroke and peripheral arterial disease (i.e. affecting the legs) – in both sexes. Some 80 per cent of all deaths among diabetics in developed countries are due to heart disease.

For women, however, the onset of diabetes has particularly serious implications as it is a considerably more powerful CHD risk factor for them than for men. An adult woman with diabetes has a risk of dying from heart disease three to seven times higher than that of a non-diabetic woman, whereas a diabetic man has a two- to four-fold increase in risk. The other bad news is that a woman over 45 is twice as likely to become a diabetic as a similarly aged man. As we shall see later, there is a very strong association between obesity and diabetes.

## CONTRIBUTORY MODIFIABLE RISK FACTORS

The following factors undoubtedly play a part in the development of CHD, although the precise level of their contribution is likely to be less than that of the major risk factors described above.

### Obesity

Obesity is nothing other than an excess of fat cells. As discussed in Action File 5, p.150, when these cells are deposited as high risk abdominal fat, they make the body much more resistant to the effects of insulin, causing the levels of insulin in the blood to rise. Raised insulin, in turn, is linked to hypertension, abnormal blood lipids (raised triglycerides and reduced HDL-C) and an increase in blood sugar levels. *Thus obesity increases heart attack risk primarily through raised insulin levels and its association with other well-known risk factors.*

But does excess weight make any *independent* contribution to CHD risk? In other words, if you are overweight but your blood pressure, cholesterol and other lipids are normal and you are non-diabetic, are you still at increased risk of heart disease? The answer appears to be 'Yes' – but not by very much. Most studies show that when hypertension, raised cholesterol and other factors are taken into account, the association between obesity and CHD almost – but not quite – disappears.

More than half the adult population is overweight, with 21 per cent of women and 17 per cent of men now classified as obese (see Figure 14).

*Figure 14*  Prevalence of obesity

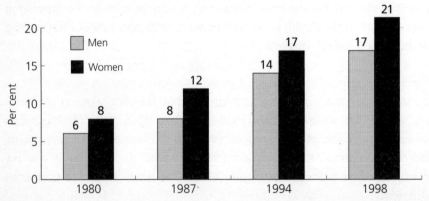

The big worry is that if these trends continue – and there is no reason to believe they won't – the health consequences in terms of hypertension, diabetes and CVD, will be extremely serious. In fact, the trend towards a reduction in heart disease referred to in Chapter 2, could well be slowed, or even reversed.

In Action File 5, p.150, we shall see that even modest weight loss can help to reduce many of the risk factors commonly associated with obesity and, by so doing, substantially reduce the risk of heart disease.

## Raised insulin levels

Insulin, as explained above, is an important causal link in the development of heart disease in women. But does insulin – apart from its associations with other well-recognised risk factors – increase the likelihood of a heart attack?

Raised insulin levels have been found in many people who do not have diabetes. Over time, many of these people will become diabetic but, even if they do not, they still appear to be prone to hypertension and heart disease. It appears that raised insulin levels may cause direct damage to the delicate cells in the endothelium (arterial lining of the arteries), making them more susceptible to plaque formation and thrombosis. Hence blood insulin levels may, in their own right, represent an important early warning sign for diabetes and CVD. Furthermore, there is evidence to suggest that high insulin levels in childhood persist into adulthood where they are associated with obesity, hypertension, raised cholesterol and triglyceride levels and, consequently, an increased risk of CHD.

The difficulty is that because of the strong association between insulin and other CHD risk factors, it is quite difficult to assess whether insulin makes a truly *independent* contribution to risk. Some preliminary studies suggest that it does *not*, but recent research is more convincing and points towards the possibility that measuring blood insulin levels may soon become one of the standard tests to evaluate a person's risk of developing diabetes and heart disease.

## Homocysteine

In many ways heart disease is considered to be a consequence of inactivity and excess: too many calories, too much fatty food, too many cigarettes and too little exercise characterise the person at high risk of heart attack. But another area which has attracted attention in recent years is the possibility that heart disease could be due, at least in part, to a vitamin deficiency.

Homocysteine is a normal breakdown product of dietary protein. There is now a growing body of evidence to suggest that homocysteine can cause damage to the endothelial lining of the arteries and may also promote movement of harmful LDL-C particles into the arterial wall, increasing the risk of plaque formation and thrombosis. Studies have shown that raised blood levels of homocysteine are associated with an increased risk of CVD, a risk comparable to conventional or classical risk factors such as smoking, high cholesterol and raised blood pressure.

Homocysteine levels are usually kept at a safe level by vitamins B6, B12 and folic acid which play a key role in breaking it down in the body. When these vitamins are lacking, homocysteine levels rise, along with the risk of heart attack and stroke. Fortunately, several studies have shown that taking these vitamins can normalise raised blood homocysteine levels.

Given that as many as one in five adults has high enough homocysteine levels to increase their risk of heart disease, the question is whether these individuals should be identified through routine testing and then given vitamin supplements.

Despite the impressive body of evidence linking homocysteine to heart disease, doctors have yet to recommend widespread testing because several key issues remain unresolved. First, no clinical trial has yet demonstrated that vitamin B supplements will truly prevent angina or heart attacks. In addition, scientists have not yet pinpointed the exact combination of vitamins that should be given to those with raised homocysteine levels. Secondly, about 30 per cent of people with high homocysteine levels do not have low levels of the key B vitamins. For them, nutritional intervention is unlikely to make any difference whatsoever. And finally, it is still unclear at what level homocysteine should be regarded as being 'high' and at what level treatment should begin.

At present there are seven major trials underway in North America, Europe and Australia, which should help to answer some of these questions. In the meantime, measuring homocysteine levels might make sense for young people with a strong family history of CVD, or for those who have suffered a heart attack in the absence of the standard risk factors that might have predicted such an event. For more information about homocysteine, vitamin supplements and how to ensure your diet is high in folate and B vitamins, see Part III, pp.216–218.

### Fibrinogen

In Chapter 1 we saw that plaque formation may be followed by a thrombosis. The blood clotting mechanism is a complex one involving the

*Figure 15*  The blood clotting mechanism

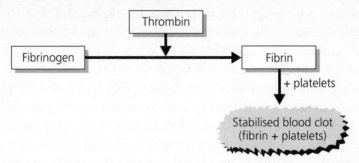

interaction of two proteins in the blood, thrombin and fibrinogen. Essentially, thrombin converts fibrinogen into a stable blood clot, which consists of fibrin and tiny particles called platelets (see Figure 15). Fibrin is subsequently broken down in the body by a process called fibrinolysis.

Given the key role of fibrinogen in the normal clotting process, it will come as no surprise that high levels increase the tendency to thrombosis. A number of studies have shown that a raised blood fibrinogen level, like a high cholesterol level, is an important independent risk factor for a heart attack in both sexes. In women, raised fibrinogen levels increase the risk of heart attack by around 70 per cent and a similar increase (80 per cent) is seen in men.

## Vitamins E, C and beta-carotene

The build-up of fatty deposits in the arteries may begin when oxygen free radicals (oxidants) interact with LDL-C (the 'bad' cholesterol). Certain vitamins, notably vitamins E, C and beta-carotene, are naturally occurring antioxidants which could prevent or reduce the oxidation of LDL-C, thereby lowering the risk of heart disease. For the three antioxidant candidates, the evidence is currently strongest for vitamin E (tocopherol).

Two large studies have examined the relationship between heart disease and vitamin E intake (from both dietary sources and vitamin supplements) and they have produced conflicting results. In the Nurses Health Study, carried out in the USA, there was a reduction in CHD risk of 40 per cent in those taking vitamin E supplements for more than two years, but no benefit from dietary vitamin E intake. In the Iowa Women's Health Study, on the other hand, the reverse was the case; women who consumed large amounts of vitamin E in *food* sources had a 64 per cent lower CHD risk than those with a low dietary intake, but there was no benefit from vitamin supplements containing vitamin E. Why there should be this apparent contradiction is unclear. In yet another study carried out in Cambridge involving subjects who already had established heart disease, administration of vitamin E supplements was found to reduce the risk of a fatal heart attack by more than a half and the risk of a non-fatal attack by 77 per cent.

Despite these findings, there are still many unanswered questions about the routine use of vitamin E and its role in prevention. For example, it is not yet clear what dosage of vitamin E is optimal in terms of CHD prevention and whether this needs to be different in those who already have evidence of heart problems compared with those who do not. In an effort to address these and other issues, several major trials – some including women – are currently underway. Results from these studies will inform future recommendations on the use of vitamin E in CVD prevention. To find out more about antioxidants and supplements, see Part III, pp.216–218.

## Alcohol consumption

You will probably have heard a great deal about the beneficial effects of alcohol, so in a section on risk factors one might be tempted to think that the risk would be one of *insufficient* alcohol, rather than the reverse! But, as I feel sure you will have gathered by now, things in the risk factor business are never that straightforward.

But let's start with some good news. Although the evidence is not entirely consistent, there is now a large body of research to suggest that moderate alcohol intake is associated with a 30–50 per cent *lower* risk of heart disease – at least in women over 50. Furthermore, despite the claims made by some producers that red wine has additional protective properties, the scientific evidence suggests that *all* alcoholic drinks are linked with a lower risk of heart disease.

The bad news is that *excessive* consumption of alcohol is associated with a number of well-known health hazards, including certain cancers, cirrhosis of the liver, stroke, road traffic accidents, suicide and violent deaths. Alcohol misuse costs society some £2.7 billion a year, of which about £164 million falls on the National Health Service. Between nine million and 15 million working days are lost each year through alcohol-related illness.

We shall be discussing safe-drinking limits in Action File 6, p.175, but for the present it is useful to recall that in December 1995, the UK Government changed the safe limit drinking guidelines for women from 14 units per week to two to three units per day (effectively up to 21 units per week). The revised guidelines were widely reported in the media and resulted in a widespread public perception that women could safely drink

*Figure 16*  Average weekly alcohol consumption in women. Note increase in 1996 in all age groups.*

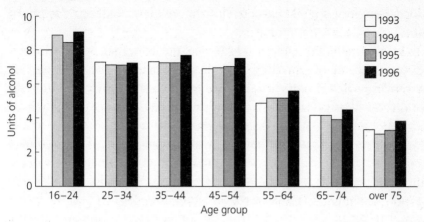

*Source:* Health Survey for England, 1996.

21 units per week. In the following year, 1996, the Health Survey for England reported an increase in average alcohol consumption among women, compared with 1993–1995 levels (see Figure 16). Moreover, the largest increase was in younger women, for whom the benefits are far less clear.

## Oral contraception, the menopause and hormone replacement therapy (HRT)

The impact of hormones on a woman's risk of cardiovascular disease is covered in Chapter 7. For now, the key 'headlines' are:

- The excess risk of a heart attack in women who use the Pill is very small and largely confined to smokers over the age of 35.
- Despite a widespread perception to the contrary, the advent of the menopause is not associated with a rise in death rates from heart disease.
- Use of HRT in post-menopausal women may not protect against heart disease.

## C-reactive protein

Heart attacks are not really that surprising when they occur in people who smoke, have high blood pressure, raised cholesterol levels or other major coronary risk factors. But some heart attacks occur in people who have no obvious risk factors – leaving the unlucky patients and their families to wonder what could have gone wrong. However, recent research is beginning to identify additional factors, which may help to provide answers in these cases and one 'hot' new risk factor for heart disease may be inflammation.

When a person has a cut or infection of the skin, the effects of inflammation – redness and swelling – are usually obvious. These changes are not produced by the skin itself, but by special chemicals released from the blood that help to resist infection and repair damaged tissues. However, a similar process may also occur inside the arteries, particularly in and around areas of plaque formation, which is the hallmark of coronary disease (see Chapter 1). The recognition that arterial damage is a dynamic process, involving cycles of damage and repair, has led to the idea that it might be possible to measure the 'inflammatory process', i.e. the body's attempt to repair damage and ward off other threats. However, inflammation may not merely indicate how much active plaque formation is taking place in the arterial wall, it may itself accelerate the entire process leading to arterial blockage. Today it is possible to measure the inflammatory response by means of a simple blood test known as the C-reactive protein (CRP) test.

Several studies have shown that high blood levels of CRP are associated with an increased risk of cardiovascular events in both men and women. Presumably, this is because individuals with higher CRP levels have a greater amount of damage and repair going on inside their arteries. In a recent report, women with the highest CRP levels had a risk of heart attack and stroke seven times higher than those with the lowest. This report, along with others, confirms that arterial damage and plaque formation are not simply plumbing problems, but a highly complex process involving cycles of damage and repair. Although more research is required, CRP looks to be yet another promising means of identifying those at increased risk of heart disease. The evidence for CRP may also explain why it is that aspirin – a powerful anti-inflammatory drug – is of benefit in preventing heart attacks. In future, patients with high CRP levels may be recommended to start taking aspirin in early adulthood.

## Stress

The subject of stress is discussed in detail in Action Plan 7, p.187, but here are the summary 'headlines':

- Stress is difficult to quantify and there is no clear association between stress levels and the risk of heart disease.

- Nowadays, attention is focussed upon a much wider range of psychosocial factors – including mental health, social and economic status, ethnicity and educational attainment – which may influence the risk of heart disease.
- The mechanisms by which these factors may influence heart attack risk are largely unknown.
- Individuals who already have heart disease may be at increased risk of further heart problems if subjected to stressful life events.
- It is not known whether stress management or other forms of psychosocial therapy, can reduce the risk of cardiovascular disease in women.

To conclude this chapter, let's now summarise the main CHD risk factors, their relationship to heart disease and the strength of the association (see Table 3 below).

*Table 3*   The main CHD risk factors

| Risk factor | Association with CHD risk | Strength |
|---|---|---|
| Age | Risk increases with age | ++++ |
| Gender | Risk generally higher in men | ++++ |
| Family history | Increased risk if father or brother with heart disease under age 55, and/or mother or sister under age 65 | ++++ |
| Polycystic Ovarian Syndrome (PCOS) | Genetic condition which may increase CHD risk by as much as seven times. Requires specialist management | +++ |
| Cigarette-smoking | Overall threefold increase in heart attack risk | ++++ |
| Hypertension (high blood pressue) | A rise of 10 mmHg in either SBP or DBP, increases heart risks by 20–30% | +++ |
| *Lipids* | | |
| Blood cholesterol (Total and LDL-C) | Increased levels increase risk: a rise of 1% increases CHD risk by 2–3% | +++ |
| HDL- cholesterol | Low levels increase risk: a change of 0.25 mmol/L can increase or decrease risk by 40–50% | +++ |
| Triglycerides | Raised levels increase risk by up to 40% | ++ |
| Physical inactivity | A physically active lifestyle can halve the risk of CHD | +++ |
| Diabetes | Diabetes increases heart attack risk in women three to seven times | ++++ |

| Risk factor | Association with CHD risk | Strength |
|---|---|---|
| Obesity | Excess body weight increases risk of heart disease – mainly by association with other risk factors | +++ |
| Insulin resistance | Increased insulin levels may increase CHD risk | + |
| Homocysteine | High levels associated with increased CHD risk | + |
| Fibrinogen | Increased levels associated with increased risk of heart attack | ++ |
| Antioxidants (Vitamins E, C and beta-carotene) | Low levels may increase risk, supplements may decrease risk | + |
| Alcohol | Moderate intake may reduce heart attack risk by 30–50% | ++ |
| *Hormones* | | |
| Oral contraceptives | No association, other than for smokers aged 35 and over | — |
| Menopause | Not associated with increased CHD rates | — |
| HRT | Reduced risk from HRT therapy not yet confirmed | ? |
| C- reactive protein | Increased levels may indicate active plaque formation and increased CHD risk | + |
| Stress and psychosocial factors | Relationship to CHD unclear, but may increase risk in those with established heart disease | ? |

Key:
++++  Very strong
+++   Strong
++    Moderate
+     Weak/Preliminary
?     Possible association
—     No association

# 4

# Heart risk appraisal – know your healthy heart numbers!

We have seen how various individual risk factors are associated with heart disease. In practice, however, these factors do not exist in isolation but interact with each other, either increasing or decreasing the overall risk as the case may be. But exactly how do these factors interrelate? For example, does a woman with a high cholesterol level but normal blood pressure run the same risk as a woman with a low cholesterol count and high blood pressure? How do risk factor levels influence the risk of heart disease in younger, compared with older women? How does each individual's risk compare with that of the average person? And how should people prioritise efforts to reduce risk in the most effective way?

These and similar questions have led to the development of Heart Risk Appraisals – methods of predicting an individual's risk of a heart attack several years into the future, based on an assessment of current risk factor levels. Traditionally, doctors have tended to use 'rules of thumb' (what amounted to little more than an informed guess) to estimate a patient's risk and to develop treatment strategies. But today, thanks to long-term research projects such as the Framingham Heart Study (p.28), mathematical models now exist which can help to make predictions more precise. Using these models, doctors are able to identify those who are at highest risk of heart disease and to target them for intensive preventive action.

When people have a clear idea of what their own risks are, they are often much more motivated to make the necessary changes in diet, exercise and other lifestyle practices, to improve their health prospects. This chapter gives you the opportunity to check your own heart risks by using a Heart Risk Appraisal (HRA) based on the work of Framingham Heart Study.

- Women who have never been diagnosed with angina or a previous heart attack should use Heart Risk Appraisal 1 (HRA1)
- Women who have been diagnosed with angina or have had a heart attack should use Heart Risk Appraisal 2 (HRA 2)

## Heart Risk Appraisal (HRA 1) for Women WITHOUT Heart Disease

Date / /

**STEP 1** Circle points for Age, Cholesterol, Blood Pressure and Other Risk Factors

| AGE | Points |
|---|---|
| 30 | -12 |
| 31 | -11 |
| 32 | -9 |
| 33 | -8 |
| 34 | -6 |
| 35 | -5 |
| 36 | -4 |
| 37 | -3 |
| 38 | -2 |
| 39 | -1 |
| 40 | 0 |
| 41 | 1 |
| 42-43 | 2 |
| 44 | 3 |
| 45-46 | 4 |
| 47-48 | 5 |
| 49-50 | 6 |
| 51-52 | 7 |
| 53-55 | 8 |
| 56-60 | 9 |
| 61-67 | 10 |
| 68-74 | 11 |

### CHOLESTEROL

| Total Cholesterol (TC) | Points | HDL-Cholesterol (HDL-C) | Points |
|---|---|---|---|
| 3.60-3.90 | -3 | 2.26-2.50 | -7 |
| 3.91-4.30 | -2 | 2.01-2.25 | -6 |
| 4.31-4.70 | -1 | 1.90-2.00 | -5 |
| 4.71-5.15 | 0 | 1.72-1.89 | -4 |
| 5.16-5.66 | 1 | 1.56-1.71 | -3 |
| 5.67-6.19 | 2 | 1.44-1.55 | -2 |
| 6.20-6.79 | 3 | 1.30-1.43 | -1 |
| 6.80-7.46 | 4 | 1.20-1.29 | 0 |
| 7.47-8.14 | 5 | 1.10-1.19 | 1 |
| 8.15-8.53 | 6 | 1.00-1.09 | 2 |
| | | 0.91-0.99 | 3 |
| | | 0.85-0.90 | 4 |
| | | 0.76-0.84 | 5 |
| | | 0.69-0.75 | 6 |
| | | 0.65-0.68 | 7 |

### BLOOD PRESSURE

| Systolic | Points |
|---|---|
| 98-104 | -2 |
| 105-112 | -1 |
| 113-120 | 0 |
| 121-129 | 1 |
| 130-139 | 2 |
| 140-149 | 3 |
| 150-160 | 4 |
| 161-172 | 5 |
| 173-185 | 6 |

| OTHER RISK FACTORS | Points |
|---|---|
| If Diabetic | 6 |
| Cigarette smoker | 4 |
| Alcohol (1 - 14 units per week) | -1 |

**STEP 2** Add up points for all risk factors (subtract minus points)

| | Points |
|---|---|
| AGE | |
| TC | |
| HDL-C | |
| BP | |
| DIABETIC | |
| CIGARETTES | |
| ALCOHOL | |
| TOTAL | |

**STEP 3** Look up points to find corresponding risk

| Points | 10-year risk % | 10-year risk level |
|---|---|---|
| ≤1 | < 2% | Very Low |
| 2 | 2% | |
| 3 | 2% | |
| 4 | 2% | |
| 5 | 3% | |
| 6 | 3% | |
| 7 | 4% | |
| 8 | 4% | Low |
| 9 | 5% | |
| 10 | 6% | |
| 11 | 6% | |
| 12 | 7% | |
| 13 | 8% | |
| 14 | 9% | |
| 15 | 10% | Moderate |
| 16 | 12% | |
| 17 | 13% | |
| 18 | 14% | |
| 19 | 16% | High |
| 20 | 18% | |
| 21 | 19% | |
| 22 | 21% | |
| 23 | 23% | |
| 24 | 25% | |
| 25 | 27% | |
| 26 | 29% | Very High |
| 27 | 31% | |
| 28 | 33% | |
| 29 | 36% | |
| 30 | 38% | |
| 31 | 40% | |
| 32 | 42% | |

**STEP 4** Compare to average 10-year risk

| Age | 10-year probability |
|---|---|
| 30-34 | < 2% |
| 35-39 | < 2% |
| 40-44 | 2% |
| 45-49 | 5% |
| 50-54 | 8% |
| 55-59 | 12% |
| 60-64 | 13% |
| 65-69 | 13% |
| 70-74 | 13% |

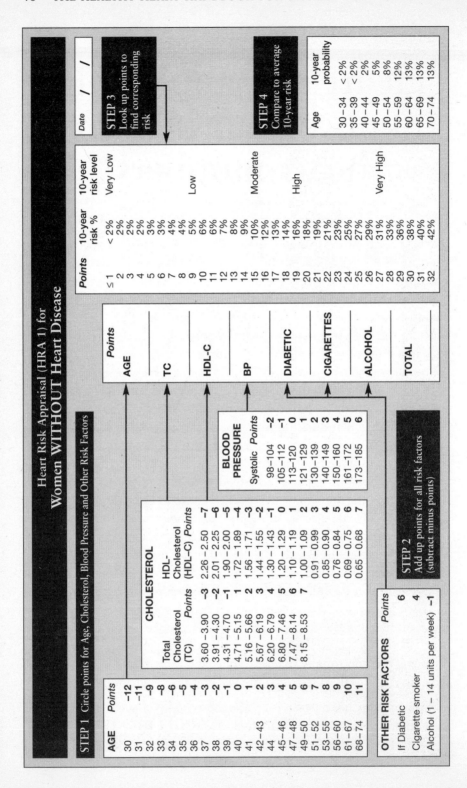

## Heart Risk Appraisal (HRA 2) for Women WITH Heart Disease

Date / /

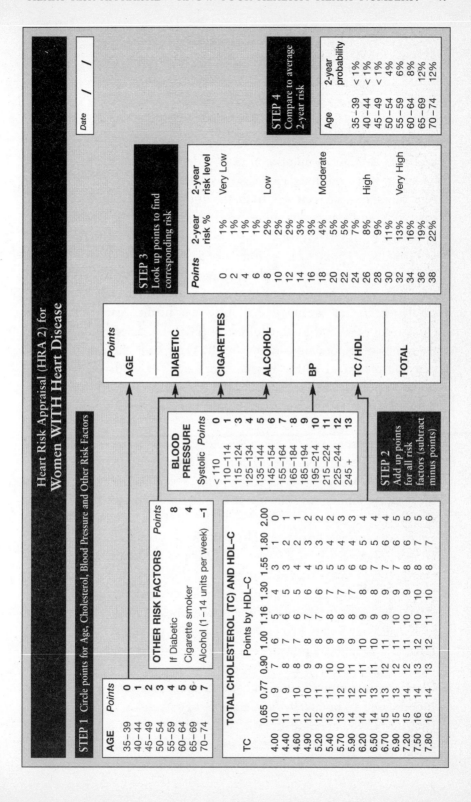

**STEP 1** Circle points for Age, Cholesterol, Blood Pressure and Other Risk Factors

| AGE | Points |
|---|---|
| 35–39 | 0 |
| 40–44 | 1 |
| 45–49 | 2 |
| 50–54 | 3 |
| 55–59 | 4 |
| 60–64 | 5 |
| 65–69 | 6 |
| 70–74 | 7 |

| OTHER RISK FACTORS | Points |
|---|---|
| If Diabetic | 8 |
| Cigarette smoker | 4 |
| Alcohol (1–14 units per week) | –1 |

**TOTAL CHOLESTEROL (TC) AND HDL-C**

TC — Points by HDL-C

| TC | 0.65 | 0.77 | 0.90 | 1.00 | 1.16 | 1.30 | 1.55 | 1.80 | 2.00 |
|---|---|---|---|---|---|---|---|---|---|
| 4.00 | 10 | 9 | 8 | 7 | 6 | 5 | 4 | 3 | 0 |
| 4.40 | 11 | 9 | 8 | 8 | 7 | 6 | 5 | 3 | 1 |
| 4.60 | 11 | 10 | 8 | 8 | 7 | 6 | 5 | 4 | 1 |
| 4.90 | 12 | 10 | 9 | 8 | 8 | 7 | 6 | 4 | 2 |
| 5.20 | 12 | 11 | 9 | 9 | 8 | 7 | 6 | 5 | 2 |
| 5.40 | 13 | 11 | 10 | 9 | 8 | 7 | 5 | 4 | 2 |
| 5.70 | 13 | 12 | 10 | 9 | 8 | 7 | 5 | 4 | 3 |
| 5.90 | 14 | 12 | 11 | 9 | 9 | 8 | 6 | 4 | 3 |
| 6.20 | 14 | 12 | 11 | 10 | 9 | 8 | 6 | 5 | 4 |
| 6.50 | 14 | 13 | 11 | 10 | 9 | 8 | 7 | 5 | 4 |
| 6.70 | 15 | 13 | 12 | 11 | 9 | 9 | 7 | 6 | 4 |
| 6.90 | 15 | 13 | 12 | 11 | 10 | 9 | 7 | 6 | 5 |
| 7.20 | 15 | 14 | 12 | 11 | 10 | 9 | 8 | 6 | 5 |
| 7.50 | 16 | 14 | 13 | 12 | 10 | 10 | 8 | 7 | 5 |
| 7.80 | 16 | 14 | 13 | 12 | 11 | 10 | 8 | 7 | 6 |

| BLOOD PRESSURE | Points |
|---|---|
| Systolic | Points |
| <110 | 0 |
| 110–114 | 1 |
| 115–124 | 3 |
| 125–134 | 4 |
| 135–144 | 5 |
| 145–154 | 6 |
| 155–164 | 7 |
| 165–184 | 8 |
| 185–194 | 9 |
| 195–214 | 10 |
| 215–224 | 11 |
| 225–244 | 12 |
| 245 + | 13 |

**STEP 2** Add up points for all risk factors (subtract minus points)

| | Points |
|---|---|
| AGE | ___ |
| DIABETIC | ___ |
| CIGARETTES | ___ |
| ALCOHOL | ___ |
| BP | ___ |
| TC/HDL | ___ |
| TOTAL | ___ |

**STEP 3** Look up points to find corresponding risk

| Points | 2-year risk % | 2-year risk level |
|---|---|---|
| 0 | 1% | Very Low |
| 2 | 1% | |
| 4 | 1% | |
| 6 | 1% | |
| 8 | 2% | Low |
| 10 | 2% | |
| 12 | 2% | |
| 14 | 3% | |
| 16 | 3% | |
| 18 | 4% | Moderate |
| 20 | 5% | |
| 22 | 5% | |
| 24 | 7% | High |
| 26 | 8% | |
| 28 | 9% | |
| 30 | 11% | Very High |
| 32 | 13% | |
| 34 | 16% | |
| 36 | 19% | |
| 38 | 22% | |

**STEP 4** Compare to average 2-year risk

| Age | 2-year probability |
|---|---|
| 35–39 | < 1% |
| 40–44 | < 1% |
| 45–49 | < 1% |
| 50–54 | 4% |
| 55–59 | 6% |
| 60–64 | 8% |
| 65–69 | 12% |
| 70–74 | 12% |

# HRA: the four steps

There are four steps in each HRA. Work through each one, following the instructions below.

## Step 1

In this first step there are six risk factors, for each of which you award yourself, or subtract, a number of points, depending on the results. The risk factors, with additional explanations where necessary, are as follows:

- **Age:** Simply select your age from the appropriate list and record the corresponding number of points for this category in the Points column near Step 2. In HRA1, for example, a woman of 31 years of age gets −11 (minus 11) points, but a woman of 51 years has +7 points (plus 7). In HRA2, the age range is slightly different in that it starts at 35. If you are 38 you get 0 points, but if you are 65, award yourself +6 points.
- **Cholesterol:** This is subdivided into two further categories: Total cholesterol (TC) and HDL-cholesterol (HDL-C). Select your TC level from the corresponding column. In HRA1, if your cholesterol is 4.50 you will record −1 in the Points column, but if 6.50 you will write down +4 points. Then select your HDL-C level and record your points. If your HDL-C is 0.95 record +3 points, but if the level is 2.00 you will record −5.

  *Note*: Those using HRA2 are given a single point score for cholesterol and HDL-C combined. For example, if your cholesterol is 5.40 and your HDL-C is 1.20, you select the points score from where the values for these two measures coincide; in this example you would give yourself +8 points. Select the value for TC and HDL-C which is closest to your own. In the above example, your HDL-C is 1.20, which, in the table, lies between HDL-C values of 1.16 and 1.30; however, it is closest to 1.16 so this is the one you use.
- **Blood pressure:** For this you need to take the systolic blood pressure (SBP), which is the higher figure of the blood pressure readings. In HRA1, if your SBP is 110 you get −1, but if 160 you get +4 points. In HRA2, if your blood pressure is 150 you get +6 points, but if 110, you receive only +1 point.
- **Cigarette smoking:** If you smoke one or more cigarette per week, allocate yourself +4 points. If you are a non- or ex-smoker you get 0 points.
- **Diabetes:** If you are diabetic, whether treated with insulin or with diet and/or drugs, allocate yourself +6 points in HRA1 and +8 points in HRA2. If you are not diabetic you get 0 points.

- **Alcohol consumption:** If you drink moderately (up to 14 units/week), give yourself –1 point. If you are teetotal, or drink more than 14 units/week, give yourself 0 points.

## Step 2

Simply add up all the plus and minus points from Step 1 to give an overall number of points.

## Step 3

Look up the predicted 10-year risk level (%) corresponding to your total number of points. If you already have evidence of heart disease, you should look up the corresponding two-year risks in HRA2. You can see how your overall risk is classified, i.e. Very Low, Low, Moderate, High and Very High.

## Step 4

In this final step you can compare your own 10-year risk (or two-year risk if you are using HRA2) with those of the average person of your age. So, for example, if your overall 10-year risk is 12 per cent and you are 55 years old, you can see that the average risk for a woman of your age is also 12 per cent. This is classified as Moderate in the overall risk level. But if your risk is 24 per cent, this is twice the average, and is classified as High.

*Note:* These HRAs provide you with an estimate of your chances of developing heart problems (or having a further heart problem), in terms of *absolute risk*. It is important to understand what this means. If, for example, you have a 10-year absolute risk of 9 per cent, this means that among a group of 100 people the same age as you, with risk factor levels (cholesterol, blood pressure etc) identical with your own, nine can be expected to develop heart problems within the next 10 years and, by implication, 91 will not. Similarly, if your estimated 10-year risk is 40 per cent, it means that among 100 people of the same age with your characteristics, 40 will develop heart problems during the next 10 years (and 60 will not).

## HRA measurements

As you can see, to complete the HRA you will need the following measurements:

- Total cholesterol (mmol/L)
- HDL-cholesterol (mmol/L)
- Blood pressure (mm Hg)

If you have had tests for heart problems, these measurements will have been done already. If not, it is best to make an appointment with your family doctor or, more easily, the practice nurse. Nowadays many practice nurses will arrange these tests for you without having to see the doctor at all. If they seem reluctant to help, don't be afraid to insist. These are important numbers which have significant implications for your future health, so don't take no for an answer! (See Action File 2, p.110, for more information about cholesterol testing.)

Most pharmacy outlets can check your blood pressure, often using automated electronic instruments rather than the more familiar mercury sphygmomanometer which you will have seen on your GP's desk. Some pharmacists also offer cholesterol testing.

## Some Examples

Here are a few examples of the HRAs in practice.

### Example 1: HRA1

In Step 1, a 65-year-old woman without heart disease earns +10 points for her age, +2 points for a TC of 5.16 and +7 for an HDL-C of 0.68. She smokes cigarettes (+4 points) and has a systolic BP of 136 (+2 points). She is also teetotal (0 points) and is a non-diabetic (0 points).

In Step 2, she adds up the points and finds they total 25. In Step 3, she finds that 25 points correspond to an estimated 10-year risk of 27 per cent. This means that among 100 women of the same age and with the same measurements, 27 will develop some evidence of heart disease within 10 years. Her overall 10-year risk level is classed as High. In Step 4 she learns she has almost twice the risk of developing heart disease compared with the average 65-year-old woman (13 per cent 10-year predicted risk).

*Comment*: Although this woman has a high risk of heart disease, her risk profile could easily be improved. If she could increase her HDL-C to 0.90 and stop smoking, this alone would reduce her points total by 7, down to 18. As a result her 10-year risk would fall to 14 per cent. In other words, by making quite modest changes in just two risk factors, she is able to halve her risk.

### Example 2: HRA1

In Step 1, a 38-year-old woman without heart disease collects –2 points for her age, +6 points for a TC of 7.60 and –6 points for an HDL-C of 2.20. Her SBP is 117 (0 points) and she is a non-smoker (0 points) and a non-diabetic (0 points), but drinks 10 units of alcohol per week (–1 point).

In Step 2 she adds up these points and finds they total –3 (6 plus points and 9 minus points). In Step 3 she finds that –3 points corresponds to a 10-year risk of less than 2 per cent. (*Note*: There are no minus point scores under the Total Points column, but clearly –3 is less than 1, and scores less than 1 point show a 10-year risk of less than 2 per cent). This places her in the very low risk category. In Step 4 she learns that the average 10-year risk for a 38-year-old woman is less than 2 per cent.

*Comment*: This is a good example of how risk factors interact with each other to produce a result which is perhaps unexpected. On first sight a total cholesterol of 7.6 mmol/L might be expected to increase risk substantially, but because there is also a high level of the protective HDL-C at 2.2 mmol/L and a good BP reading, the overall risk is very low.

### Example 3:  HRA2
In Step 1, a 55-year-old woman with diabetes and a previous history of a heart attack and angina, receives +4 points for her age and a further +8 points for diabetes. A total cholesterol concentration of 7.49 and an HDL-C of 0.77 earns another +14 points and her cigarette smoking another +4 points. Her SBP is 128 (+4 points) and her alcohol consumption is heavy – around 50 units per week for which she receives 0 points.

In Step 2 she adds up these points and finds they total 34. In Step 3 she finds that 34 points corresponds to a two-year risk of 16 per cent which means that of 100 women of the same age, with the same history and current measurements, 16 will have a further heart attack during the next two years. In terms of her overall risk level, she is in the Very High category. In Step 4 she discovers that the average 55-year-old woman with heart disease has a 2-year risk of a further cardiac problem of 6 per cent. In other words, her own risk is two-and-a-half times the average.

*Comment*: This woman already has coronary disease and has a high risk of suffering another heart attack during the next two years. However, by stopping smoking and reducing her cholesterol to 5.9, increasing her HDL-C to 1.0 and by moderating her alcohol intake to less than 14 units per week (for which she then receives –1), she can reduce her points total to 24, which equates to a two-year risk of just 7 per cent – close to the average of 6 per cent for a woman of her age with a history of heart disease. This again demonstrates that very modest changes in risk factors can result in very significant reductions in risk – in this case by 56 per cent.

## Some notes and a caveat

Please note the following when using the HRAs:

- Relatively small changes in multiple factors have a much greater impact on risk than large changes in a single risk factor.
- Some risk factors have not been included in these HRAs – notably body weight, a family history of heart disease and physical activity. This does not mean that these are not important in terms of heart risks, only that they are difficult to quantify in any one individual.
- The charts must only be used for the age ranges given.

The caveat is that while risk prediction can be a valuable tool in prevention, no mathematical model can hope to capture all the factors that influence health and disease. The Framingham scores are based on studies of populations; using the results to predict outcomes in *individuals* is very different. Having a high risk score does not mean that you will develop problems, only that you are more likely to.

*Note*: **These tables, and the risk scores they provide, should not be taken as 100 per cent reliable. They are merely meant to offer general guidelines and a basis for action.**

# 5
# Diagnosis and treatment

When doctors talk about prevention, they often distinguish between 'primary prevention' i.e. trying to prevent heart disease from developing in the first place and 'secondary prevention', trying to avoid further problems in those who have already suffered a heart attack or who have angina. Most of what is said in this book, particularly with respect to risk factors, is applicable to both primary and secondary prevention. But this chapter is specifically for those of you who have already suffered a heart attack, undergone heart surgery, or who have other symptoms of heart disease such as angina. Although having a previous history of heart disease undoubtedly increases your risks in the future, the good news is that aggressive modification of risk factors, combined with modern drug therapy, can greatly improve your chances of living a normal life and avoiding any further problems.

Because of your symptoms you may have undergone (or have to undergo) special diagnostic tests to establish the extent of your heart problems and, more importantly, what form of treatment would be most appropriate. In addition, you may have been prescribed specific drugs for angina, hypertension or lowering cholesterol etc, and these also have to be considered as key components in an overall strategy for secondary prevention. The practical side of modifying risk factors (covered in detail in Part II) is really no different for you compared with someone who does not have heart disease; it is simply that you have even more incentive to make and maintain appropriate lifestyle changes.

So, the aim in this chapter is to:

1. Provide a brief overview of the diagnostic tests you may be asked to undertake by your doctor.
2. Describe the most common forms of surgical treatment for heart disease.
3. Provide some basic information on the drugs most commonly used in the treatment of heart disease, including angina, hypertension and disturbed heart rhythms.

# Diagnostic tests

There are several commonly used tests for the diagnosis of CHD. Of these the electrocardiogram (ECG) is pretty standard for anyone with symptoms of heart disease. Whether or not you have the others will depend on the ECG results and a number of other factors. Most of these tests are carried out in hospital as a day case (which means you do not have to stay in overnight).

## Electrocardiogram (ECG)

There are two types of electrocardiogram, or ECG: resting and exercise. As the term implies, the resting ECG records the rhythm and electrical activity of the heart at rest. The test is painless and usually takes just a few minutes. Small adhesive patches are put on your arms, chest and legs and are connected to a recording instrument. The ECG tracing, which essentially comes out as a series of spikes and waves, is then taken. If you have coronary disease, the ECG may show certain abnormalities. However, it is possible to have heart disease even in the presence of a normal ECG, which is why your doctor may also suggest an exercise ECG.

An exercise ECG is carried out while you are exercising – usually walking on a treadmill or pedalling a stationary exercise bicycle. During strenuous exercise, the heart has to work five times harder than it does at rest and it must be able to get oxygen-rich blood to the heart muscle. As we saw in Chapter 1, if the coronary arteries are narrowed, they may be unable to allow enough blood through to the heart – a condition referred to by doctors as *ischaemia*. An ECG taken at this point may show a clearly abnormal pattern and there may also be changes in the rhythm of the heart and blood pressure. However, it is a safe test and very rarely associated with any serious complications. The doctor and technician carrying out the test will monitor the ECG, heart rhythm and blood pressure closely and the test will usually be discontinued when you have achieved the required heart rate. For reasons that need not concern us here, the exercise ECG is often more difficult to interpret in a woman than in a man. Nevertheless, in experienced hands it is still a useful tool in the investigation of chest pain and other heart-associated symptoms in women.

## Radioactive isotope tests

These tests make use of a very small and harmless amount of radioactive material (isotope) which is injected into the bloodstream while the patient is exercising on a treadmill or bicycle. The isotope (usually thallium or technetium) is taken up by the heart muscle and emits rays which can then be picked up by a special camera positioned close to the chest. The principle of the test is that the areas of the heart which have a poor blood supply are unable to take up the isotope as well as the rest of the heart muscle. These areas of 'underperfusion' can then be seen on the images produced by the camera, providing valuable information about the location and extent of any coronary arterial narrowing. The test may also be used to study the heart in people who can't manage the treadmill or bicycle, for example because of arthritis or lung disease.

Because of the cost, only about three or four in every 100 people with suspected heart disease have an isotope test. In women it can often be more useful than the exercise ECG for diagnosing angina.

## Echocardiography

Echocardiography is the name given to an investigation which uses sound beams to take pictures of the heart. With this type of scanner (the same instrument which takes pictures of the baby in the mother's womb) it is possible to see the heart muscle contracting and to identify areas that are contracting poorly because of poor blood supply from the coronary arteries. It is also useful for identifying other forms of heart disease, including cardiomyopathy (a genetic form of heart muscle disease) and disease of the heart valves.

Although usually carried out at rest, some centres now have the ability to perform stress echocardiography. In principle it is similar to the isotope test, except that sound-waves rather than radioactivity are involved.

## Coronary angiography

Also called 'coronary arteriography' or 'coronary angiogram'. A catheter (fine hollow tube) is carefully introduced into the main artery in the groin or the forearm and gently advanced until the tip of the catheter reaches the openings of the coronary arteries. A special dye is then injected into the coronary arteries and X-rays are taken from various angles. These will show a 'road map' of your coronary arteries and, in particular, the location and extent of any arterial narrowing. Based on this information, the doctor can then decide what (if any) treatment is required. The test is performed under local anaesthetic so the patient is fully conscious throughout.

There are four possible results from your angiography:

1. Your disease can be treated with angioplasty.
2. Your disease is best treated with coronary artery bypass grafting (CABG).
3. You are suitable for either angioplasty or surgery.
4. Surgery and angioplasty are not indicated.

These treatment options are discussed later.

## Other tests

Several other sophisticated investigations using different imaging methods are currently under development. While not routinely used at present, they may well become standard tests in future.

### Magnetic Resonance Imaging (MRI)

MRI is a remarkable diagnostic tool that uses magnets rather than X-rays or sound waves to create three-dimensional images of internal organs. It is already routinely used in the investigation of many diseases, particularly those involving the brain or skeleton. The problem in imaging the heart, of course, is that, unlike the brain or skeleton, it is a moving structure and this poses particular technical difficulties. Nevertheless, MRI may one day replace coronary angiography as the routine test for assessing the location and extent of coronary artery disease.

### Positron Emission Tomography (PET)

PET is a relatively new research instrument that measures how efficient the heart muscle cells are in utilising oxygen. It is an extremely expensive test, requiring sophisticated technology which is usually only available in very large centres.

### Ultrafast CAT scanning

This is another relatively new method of visualising the coronary arteries without having to resort to cardiac catheterisation. A well established X-ray technique called computerised axial tomography (CAT) is used to image the heart. The test can identify calcium deposits in the arteries, which are usually associated with plaque formation and, thus, coronary artery disease. In addition to its use as a diagnostic tool, ultrafast CAT may also have some application as a screening tool.

# Surgical treatment

By no means everyone who has angina or a heart attack will require surgery and many patients do perfectly well on a combination of drugs and lifestyle management. However, when symptoms become severe or unresponsive to medical treatment, the results of surgery can be dramatic. Women with angina of many years' standing may suddenly be able to take up regular exercise again – indeed, some have even completed marathons! Of course, surgery does not 'cure' the underlying disease and you still need to take all the steps necessary to prevent any further deterioration in your arteries, either through lifestyle modification such as stopping smoking, or with drugs such as those used to treat high blood pressure or lower cholesterol.

There are two main forms of surgical treatment for coronary artery disease: coronary angioplasty and coronary artery bypass grafting (CABG).

## Coronary angioplasty

A coronary angiogram (see p.57) is the 'gold-standard' test for determining both the location and the degree of any narrowing in the coronary arteries. If the cardiologist feels that the disease can be treated with angioplasty, he/she will usually go ahead and perform this immediately after the arteriogram. The technique was first used in 1977 and around 23,500 angioplasties are now performed each year in the UK.

During angioplasty, a special catheter with a small inflatable balloon at its tip is introduced into the artery and passed into the narrowed segment.

*Figure 17*   Coronary angioplasty
The catheter is passed through the artery until it reaches the blockage. The sausage-shaped balloon tip is then inflated to flatten the plaque into the artery wall and improve the blood flow. The balloon is inflated to about 3mm (1/8in) in diameter.

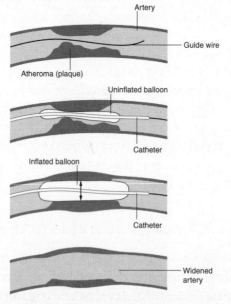

The balloon is then inflated and effectively squashes the fatty tissue responsible for the narrowing into the arterial wall (see Figure 17). The balloon is then deflated and withdrawn, leaving the artery open.

At least 90 per cent of angioplasty operations are successful. Very occasionally, however, an angioplasty may cause blockage or rupture of an artery, which will require immediate open-heart surgery. This happens, on average, in about one in every 100 cases, but the results of this emergency surgery are good.

The advantage of coronary angioplasty is that, unlike open-heart surgery, it can be done in a relatively short time and is much less traumatic. An overnight stay is all that is required and, depending upon your occupation, you can be back at work within a week. It is, however, technically demanding and may occasionally take rather longer than predicted to manipulate the balloon into exactly the right position.

The main problem with coronary angioplasty is that in about a third of cases, the narrowing returns within four to six months of the procedure. If necessary, the procedure can be repeated, but nowadays when angioplasties are performed a special support frame called a 'stent' is often inserted during the operation. The stent is a short tube of stainless steel mesh which is inserted at the part of the artery which is to be widened. As the balloon is inflated, the stent frame expands slightly to hold the artery open. The catheter is then removed, leaving the stent in place, thus hopefully preventing any re-narrowing of the artery.

Of course, angioplasty may not be appropriate for everyone. In women with disease in all three main branches of the coronary arterial system, or where there are multiple narrowings in one or more arteries, the only option may be to recommend coronary artery bypass grafting (CABG).

## Coronary artery bypass grafting (CABG)

This is major surgery, requiring a stay in hospital of five to seven days. It has been one of the major advances in the treatment of angina and is also effective in improving the outlook for patients with severe narrowing of the main coronary arteries. The first CABG procedure was carried out in 1967. Today about 25,000 CABGs are performed in the UK each year. Before any decision to operate, a coronary angiogram will be needed to identify which vessels are blocked and where the grafts are to be inserted.

### The operation

In most bypass operations the surgeon gains access to the heart by making an incision in the middle of the chest and then splitting the breastbone lengthways. While the heart is being operated on, it is necessary to stop the flow of blood through the heart and lungs. This is achieved by means of a heart-lung bypass machine, which takes over the function of the heart and lungs for the period of the operation and provides a constant supply of oxygen-rich blood to the brain and other tissues of the body.

The main aim of CABG is, as its name implies, to bypass the narrowed section of the diseased arteries. This is done by grafting a blood vessel between the aorta (the main blood vessel of the heart) and a point in the coronary artery beyond the narrowed or blocked area (see Figure 18). In some patients this may mean a single graft to one affected artery, but more commonly two, three (triple bypass) or four (quadruple bypass) grafts will be required.

The blood vessel used for the graft will come from another part of your body. For many years surgeons used leg veins for this purpose, but nowadays they are more likely to use an artery that runs down the inside of the chest wall (called the internal mammary artery). This artery is more able to withstand the relatively high pressure in the coronary arteries and is less likely to develop narrowings than vein grafts. Some patients will have a mixture of vein and arterial grafts.

*Figure 18*  **Coronary artery bypass operation**

In coronary artery bypass graft (CABG) operations, surgeons use an artery or a vein from elsewhere in the body to bypass blocked coronary arteries.

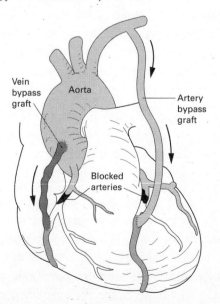

### Risks and benefits

About 80 per cent of patients who have a bypass operation experience immediate and lasting relief from angina and most of the remaining 20 per cent experience some improvement. Narrowing of the graft due to plaque occurs in about five per cent of patients every year and this is much more likely to occur if risk factors such as smoking, hypertension and cholesterol are not controlled. The risk of surgery will depend very much on the severity of the underlying disease, whether there has been a previous heart attack, the age of the patient and the presence of other risk factors, such as diabetes. Generally speaking, however, the risk of death within a month of the operation is quite low – around two per cent (20 in every 1000).

If anginal symptoms do eventually recur, a further operation may be needed, although this is obviously much more technically difficult than the first operation. This is why close attention to risk factors is so crucial. In some patients symptoms can be dealt with by a simple coronary angioplasty, or changes in medication.

## Angioplasty or CABG?

For some patients, particularly those with severe disease involving all three branches of the coronary arteries (triple vessel disease), the best option is to have CABG. This is because surgery will not only improve symptoms but is also likely to reduce the risk of a major heart attack or sudden death. For other patients with less severe disease, angioplasty may be the best option and in some centres you may be given a choice. There are advantages and disadvantages to both procedures, the most obvious one being that angioplasty avoids the need for major surgery. Your family GP and consultant surgeon will be able to advise you as to what may be the best option for you. However, in terms of the longer term outlook (three to five years) there is no major difference between these procedures.

## Keyhole surgery

Keyhole surgery for coronary heart disease is being evaluated, so it is not yet widely used in routine practice. Because it requires a smaller incision than standard CABG, the potential advantages are obvious: less bleeding, fewer serious complications and an earlier return to work. However, because only a small part of the heart is exposed, the approach is technically difficult and it will not be a suitable procedure for all patients.

## Other forms of heart surgery

Several other forms of heart surgery are currently being evaluated.

### Transmyocardial laser revascularisation (TMLR)

TMLR is a new procedure which may be of benefit for patients who are unsuitable for either CABG or angioplasty, and whose symptoms cannot be controlled by medication. After a small incision is made in the chest wall, a powerful laser is used to 'drill' a series of 30–40 holes through the heart muscle itself (not the coronary arteries). The tiny channels created in this way allow oxygen-rich blood to get to areas of the myocardium (heart muscle) which have been starved of blood because of narrowed arteries. The technique is still in the research stage and the results, while encouraging, are not yet conclusive. It is possible that TMLR will become an option for patients with severe disease, perhaps used in combination with CABG and/or angioplasty.

### Heart transplantation

For a minority of patients with advanced heart disease, the only available option may be a transplant. Remarkable progress in heart transplantation techniques has been made during the last decade, including the development of new drugs which help to prevent rejection. Today, heart transplantation is no longer regarded as an experimental procedure. Indeed, several large teaching hospitals have a busy transplantation programme, although there is always a shortage of suitable donors.

Recently, genetically engineered pig hearts have been proposed as providing an unlimited source of donor organs for those who require transplantation. However, there are many major medical and ethical questions which will have to be addressed before this becomes a viable option.

# Drug treatment

The development of drugs for the treatment of heart disease has been one of the miracles of modern science. These new drugs are effective because they are powerful. So, if you have been prescribed any of them, you should know why you are taking them, how to take them, roughly how they work and what, if any, side-effects may occur.

Each drug has one official name (the 'generic' name), but it may also be prescribed under a trade name (or 'proprietary' name) given to it by the pharmaceutical company. For example, a drug belonging to a group known as beta-blockers used to treat angina and hypertension has the generic name Atenolol and the proprietary name Tenormin.

## What are heart drugs used for?

Drugs are used to treat angina, hypertension, high blood cholesterol, heart failure, disturbances in heart rhythm and poor circulation in the legs. Other drugs may be given to thin the blood and reduce the tendency to develop thromboses (blood clots). The main forms of heart disease and the drugs used to treat them are summarized in Table 4, pp.72–74.

## How are heart drugs taken?

Drugs given for heart problems can be taken in a number of different ways:

- *Orally* The drug is taken by mouth in the form of tablets or capsules to be swallowed. (The most usual form of prescription.)
- *Sublingually* The drug is held under the tongue until it dissolves.
- *Aerosol spray* The drug is directed into the mouth by means of an aerosol spray.
- *Self-adhesive skin patches* A patch containing the drug is placed on the skin and the drug is gradually absorbed through the skin into the bloodstream.
- *Subcutaneously* The drug is injected just under the surface of the skin.
- *Intramuscularly* The drug is injected into a muscle, usually the thigh or buttock.
- *Intravenously* The drug is injected into a vein, either with a needle and syringe or through an intravenous drip.

## How do heart drugs work and what are their side-effects?

The various groups of drugs have different modes of action and potentially different side-effects. Most drugs used to treat heart disease are very safe and dangerous side-effects are extremely rare. However, minor side-effects occur fairly frequently and it is useful for you to be aware of the more common ones. The most important groups of drugs are as follows:

- ACE inhibitors
- Anti-arrhythmics
- Anticoagulants
- Aspirin and other anti-platelet drugs
- Beta-blockers
- Calcium antagonists

- Cholesterol lowering drugs
- Diuretics
- Nitrates
- Potassium channel activators

A brief description of each of these is given below, including some notes on common side-effects.

### ACE inhibitors

Angiotensin II is a blood chemical which has a powerful narrowing effect upon the blood vessels. It is produced by the actions of another chemical called 'angiotensin converting enzyme' or ACE. ACE inhibitors reduce the amount of angiotensin II in the blood, allowing coronary and other arteries to relax. By helping blood vessels to dilate, these drugs lower blood pressure and ease the heart's workload.

ACE inhibitors are now standard care for people with heart failure. (The term 'heart failure' simply means that the pumping action of the heart is inadequate for the body's requirements. It does not mean that the heart has stopped.) Recent research suggests they may also offer life-saving benefits to people with evidence of heart disease, but who do not have obvious heart failure. This is why they are sometimes prescribed for patients who have suffered a heart attack or who are at high risk from heart disease. Exactly why ACE inhibitors should be so beneficial in those without heart failure is not yet clear, although there is some evidence that they may help to make plaque more stable and, therefore, less liable to rupture. ACE inhibitors have become widely prescribed for hypertension, and diabetics may also benefit from ACE therapy.

Although ACE inhibitors are usually well tolerated, they have a number of important unwanted side-effects. For example, they may cause a marked fall in blood pressure, particularly in patients who are already taking diuretics. In addition they may cause disturbances in kidney function, which is why your doctor will want to check this with an occasional blood test. They can also cause skin rashes, nausea, breathlessness, dizziness, fatigue, headache and may affect your sense of taste. Very occasionally they may produce a major allergic reaction with swelling of the hands, face and eyes.

However, the most common side-effect is a persistent, dry, irritating cough, which is more common in women than men. This may improve by reducing the dosage, although many patients simply get used to it.

## Anti-arrhythmics

As their name implies, these drugs are used to control abnormal heart rhythms. Although beta-blockers and calcium antagonists are also used to treat heart rhythm disturbances, anti-arrhythmics are used almost exclusively for this purpose.

Amiodarone is among the most potent of the anti-arrhythmic drugs currently available. Unfortunately, however, its general usefulness is limited by the reactions it may sometimes produce. These include headache, nausea, flushing, dizziness and, more seriously, disturbances in thyroid, liver and lung function. Your doctor will wish to monitor your response to this drug, with regular blood tests and occasional chest X-rays.

Flecainide is another powerful drug used for the treatment of serious disturbances in cardiac rhythm. Like Amiodarone, it has significant side-effects, including nausea, skin rashes, eye problems and disturbances in liver and lung function.

Digoxin, or digitalis, is derived from the leaf of the common purple foxglove and has been used to treat heart problems for more than two centuries. Since its main effect is to strengthen the heart's action, it is commonly used in the treatment of heart failure. It is also effective in the treatment of a common rhythm disturbance called atrial fibrillation. This is a condition in which the heart beats rapidly but also irregularly and which may lead to heart failure. Digoxin slows the heart and improves symptoms such as breathlessness and palpitations, although it may not restore normal rhythm.

Digoxin is usually well tolerated, although it can cause loss of appetite and nausea. Less frequently, it can cause vomiting, rashes, weakness and fainting.

Apart from those mentioned above, there are several other anti-arrhythmic drugs available which have their own interactions and potential adverse side-effects. Your doctor will be able to explain which is the most appropriate for you and you should follow his/her instructions very carefully. Do please remember that these are very powerful drugs and should only be taken under close medical supervision and with continuous monitoring. If you are taking any of these tablets and experience any side-effects which seem unusual, you should contact your doctor immediately.

## Anticoagulants

A blood clot consists of two main elements: a protein called fibrin and small blood cells called platelets. Anticoagulants, as their name suggests, prevent fibrin from forming and, therefore, interfere with the normal clotting mechanisms. Because they have the effect of thinning the blood, they reduce the likelihood of any thromboses in the arteries or veins.

The most commonly prescribed oral anticoagulant for long-term treatment is Warfarin. It may be given to patients who have received artificial heart valves, but is also prescribed for those who have disturbances in heart rhythm (such as atrial fibrillation) and for patients with deep vein thromboses (clots in the leg veins) and pulmonary emboli (clots in the lungs).

Although anticoagulants are effective because of their effects on bleeding, regular blood tests are required to ensure that the thinning of the blood is at the correct level. At first, these tests will be required almost every day, but later, once the results have been stabilized, they can be carried out every six to eight weeks.

The other problem is that oral anticoagulants interact with many other medicines, including antibiotics, aspirin and some drugs used to treat arthritis, gout, epilepsy and diabetes. If you are taking anticoagulants you should always carry an Anticoagulant Card and remember to inform doctors, nurses and your dentist if you need treatment of any kind. You should also be aware of the following signs which may suggest that the dose of anticoagulant is too high:

- prolonged bleeding from cuts
- bleeding gums
- red or black urine
- prolonged nose bleeds
- red or black bowel motions
- vaginal bleeding or heavier than normal bleeding during periods

If you are worried by any of these, or other symptoms, contact your anticoagulant clinic, GP or casualty department without delay.

### Aspirin and other anti-platelet drugs
Aspirin has been used for pain relief for more than 2000 years, but it is also effective in preventing blood clotting. This it does, not by any effect on fibrin, but by reducing the 'stickiness' of platelets – the small cells which join with fibrin to form a blood clot.

Aspirin has been shown to reduce the risk of dying after a heart attack and the risk of a further attack and stroke in those who have already suffered one of these events. It is now used almost routinely in patients with known coronary heart disease, including angina, unless there are good reasons for not giving it. This is *secondary* prevention.

But should aspirin be used for *primary* prevention (i.e. to prevent heart attacks in high-risk women who do not yet have obvious coronary disease)? The difficulty in answering this question is that, although aspirin tends to protect against heart attack and the common forms of stroke, one particular form of stroke – the type that develops not because of a blockage in the artery, but because the blood vessel actually breaks and allows blood to escape into the brain itself (known as haemorrhagic stroke) – may actually be more common in women taking aspirin. Now, for women with established cardiovascular disease, the benefits of aspirin easily outweigh the risk of a haemorrhagic stroke, whereas for women without disease, the risk benefit is not so clear cut. Until better evidence is available, therefore, low-dose aspirin is *not* routinely recommended for primary prevention in high-risk women.

Aspirin can cause indigestion, nausea, vomiting and constipation, although enteric coated preparations may help to reduce the stomach problems. In susceptible individuals, aspirin may occasionally precipitate an acute attack of asthma. Women are generally cautioned against taking aspirin during pregnancy because it may increase the risk of foetal and maternal bleeding. These unwanted effects are another reason for not prescribing aspirin for those who do not have established cardiovascular disease.

Other, newer, anti-platelet drugs including Clopidogrel and Ticlopidine are currently being evaluated.

### Beta-blockers

These drugs block the action of adrenaline on the heart and blood vessels, thus slowing the heart and making it beat less forcefully. Because the heart beats at a lower rate, it demands less oxygen and, therefore, is less affected by any impairment of blood supply from narrowed coronary arteries. Beta-blockers are very effective in the treatment of angina, hypertension and some disturbances in heart rhythm. They also reduce the risk of further heart attacks in people who have already had one.

Unwanted side-effects of beta-blockers include a tendency to constrict the airways, so they should be avoided in people who suffer from asthma or wheezing. Because beta-blockers may also constrict smaller blood vessels, some patients complain of cold hands and feet. In people who are taking medication for diabetes, beta-blockers may also mask the symptoms of hypoglycaemia (low blood sugar). Other unwanted effects include fatigue, nightmares, nausea, skin rashes and dry eyes.

Because beta-blockers reduce the force of the heartbeat, they must be used with great care in patients with heart failure.

## Calcium antagonists

Muscle cells in the heart and elsewhere need a regular inflow of calcium in order to function properly. Calcium antagonists, also known as calcium channel blockers, reduce the amount of calcium entering muscle cells of the coronary and other arteries, causing them to relax. This improves blood flow through the narrowed artery and also reduces the amount of work the heart must do in order to pump blood around the body. Calcium antagonists are used in the treatment of angina (often combined with other drugs such as beta-blockers and nitrates) and hypertension. Some calcium channel blockers, such as Verapamil, are also used to treat some disorders of heart rhythm.

Verapamil and Diltiazem both cause slowing of the heart so that if they are used with beta-blockers (which also slow the heart) the combined effect may produce serious slowing of the heart, or even heart block and fainting.

Serious side-effects are uncommon with calcium antagonists, but they occasionally cause headaches, nausea, dizziness and flushing. Another annoying side effect is ankle-swelling, which may be more marked if you already have varicose veins.

## Cholesterol-lowering drugs

As we saw in Chapter 3, the collective term 'blood lipids' refers to all the fatty substances in the blood, including LDL-cholesterol, HDL-cholesterol and triglycerides. The principal aim of treatment is to lower total blood cholesterol and LDL-cholesterol in particular, but reducing triglyceride levels may also be important.

As emphasised in Action File 2, p.105, the first-line treatment for high cholesterol levels is to reduce your dietary intake of saturated fat. Some patients, and some doctors, seem to think that because modern cholesterol-lowering drugs are so powerful, they have somehow superceded the need for dietary changes. This is not true. Simply by choosing healthier foods it is possible to lower your cholesterol level by 10 per cent or even more and, whether you eventually need to take medication or not, you should always ensure that you stick to a low-fat diet to begin with. However, some people, regardless of how hard they try, are unable to get their cholesterol down to a safe level by losing weight and reducing their fat intake. They may, for example, have a genetic tendency to high blood cholesterol levels. Whatever the reason, if diet alone fails, it is then sensible to consider medication. There are several groups of drugs available, including statins, bile resins and fibrates.

Statins are cholesterol-lowering drugs which became generally available in the mid-1990s. They work by slowing the production of cholesterol in the liver and are able to reduce total cholesterol levels by 25–45 per cent and LDL-cholesterol by 30–50 per cent. Overall, statins reduce the risks of fatal and non-fatal heart attack by around 25–30 per cent. Moreover, statin treatment seems to be as effective in people in their 70s as it is in middle-aged people. Many statins have become available in recent years, but the two most commonly used are Simvastatin and Pravastatin, which are both equally effective.

Statins can occasionally produce inflammation of the liver and should not be used in people with liver disease. So, before you start taking them, your doctor will wish to carry out a blood test to make sure your liver is functioning normally and this test will be repeated at intervals while you are on treatment. Another rare side-effect of statins is *myositis* (inflammation of the muscles), which usually occurs in the first few weeks after starting treatment. If you experience pain, tenderness, or weakness in the muscles of your arms and legs, you should tell your doctor immediately. In general, however, statins are well tolerated and have few common side-effects, apart from nausea and headache. They are usually taken as a single dose at night, and the dosage is adjusted according to the effect on total and LDL-cholesterol.

Two other types of cholesterol-lowering drugs can be used if statins are not suitable. These are bile resins, which bind bile acids, and fibrates.

Bile resins – of which the main representatives are Cholestyramine and Colestipol – are not absorbed into the body, but pass unaltered through the gut. As they do so, they bind bile acids, which contain cholesterol, and excrete them in the stools. Resins have been shown to reduce the risk of heart attack by only around 10–15 per cent, so they are less potent than the statins.

Bile resins come in powder form in sachets, and usually need to be mixed with fruit juice before you take them. Because resins are not absorbed into the body, they cannot cause any serious side-effects, although some people experience a feeling of fullness when they start treatment. Other side-effects are flatulence, bloating, heartburn and constipation, but these tend to lessen with continued use.

Fibrates come in tablet or capsule form and include Bezafibrate and Gemfibrozil. They are very useful in people who have a high level of both cholesterol and triglycerides, for example, diabetics. Fibrates reduce triglycerides, increase HDL-cholesterol and lower total cholesterol, the net effect being a significant lowering of coronary risk. They are generally well tolerated and have few side-effects, the most common being nausea, rashes and headache. As with statins, they may occasionally cause muscle pain in the first few weeks of use, but this usually goes quickly when the drug is withdrawn.

## Diuretics

Diuretics, or water tablets, increase the amount of salt and water passed in the urine. As a result of this, the volume of blood in the circulation is reduced and blood pressure falls. Diuretics are, therefore, used to treat hypertension; indeed, mild hypertension can often be managed by diuretics alone. If this is not sufficient to keep the blood pressure under control, a beta-blocker is usually added. Nowadays, drugs consisting of a combination of diuretic and beta-blocker are available. Diuretics are also very effective in the treatment of heart failure.

There are several types of diuretic, some of which may result in excessive loss of potassium. Because an adequate blood level of potassium is essential for the normal functioning of the body, doctors often guard against this by prescribing a *combination* of a diuretic and a potassium supplement (indicated by the letter K, which is the chemical symbol for potassium in the brand name, for example Burinex K). Other diuretics, such as Spironolactone are 'potassium-sparing' and do not, therefore, require potassium supplements. If you are taking diuretics you should be careful not to take too much salt in your food, since this can counteract the effects of the diuretics. This means not adding salt during cooking or at the table and avoiding salty foods in general.

Some of the more important side-effects of diuretics include:

- An increase in blood sugar levels, sometimes precipitating diabetes; individuals who are already diabetic are not generally prescribed diuretics.
- A rise in blood cholesterol levels, leading to an increased risk of heart disease.
- A rise in uric acid levels leading, on rare occasions, to gout.

## Nitrates

Nitrates in various forms have been used in the treatment of angina for more than a hundred years and are the most common drugs used to treat this condition. Nitrates relax the muscle layer in the walls of the coronary arteries, making them wider and thus improving blood flow to the heart. Glyceryl Trinitrate, also called GTN or Nitroglycerine, is absorbed very quickly through the lining of the mouth and is either taken as a small tablet under the tongue, or as a spray. This makes it extremely effective at relieving acute attacks of angina. If you have an attack you should stand still or sit down and take a tablet (or spray) and if the pain is not relieved after a couple of minutes, you can take another. (Incidentally, if you use a spray you don't need to shake the canister before use.) There are also self-adhesive skin-patches containing GTN, and even an ointment form of the drug. If you use GTN tablets, you should always carry a fresh supply and keep them in an amber bottle which will prevent them from deteriorating in sunlight. You should not store them with other tablets or keep them out in a pill box.

Although nitrates work by dilating the coronary arteries, they have a similar effect on other blood vessels in the body, which can lead to unwanted side-effects, the most common of which are flushing, headache and dizziness, although these tend to become less of a problem when you have used nitrates for a while.

While GTN is the most effective form of nitrate for relief of an acute anginal attack, other longer-acting forms of nitrates (known as mononitrates and dinitrates) are also prescribed for the prevention of angina. These forms of the drug are taken by mouth, are slower to act and are taken once or twice a day. Unfortunately, they become less effective when used continuously over a long period.

## Potassium channel activators

These new drugs act in a similar way to the nitrates described above, causing relaxation of the coronary arteries and hence improved blood flow. Unlike nitrates, however, they do not appear to become less effective with continued use. Unwanted effects are similar to those of nitrates, i.e. flushing, headache, dizziness and indigestion.

Examples of all the main groups discussed above, together with their main side-effects, are summarised in Table 4.

*Table 4*  Common drugs for heart disease and their side-effects

| Class of drug | Generic name | Administration | Uses | Possible side-effects |
|---|---|---|---|---|
| ACE inhibitors | Captopril | Tablets | For treatment | Persistent dry |
| | Cilazapril | Tablets | of heart | cough, |
| | Enalapril | Tablets | failure and | dizziness, skin |
| | Fosinopril | Tablets | hypertension | rashes, nausea |
| | Imidapril | Tablets | | and headache |
| | Lisinopril | Tablets | | |
| | Perindopril | Tablets | | |
| | Quinapril | Tablets | | |
| | Ramipril | Capsules | | |
| | Trandolapril | Capsules | | |

| Class of drug | Generic name | Administration | Uses | Possible side-effects |
|---|---|---|---|---|
| Anti-arrhythmics | Amiodarone<br>Digoxin<br>Disopyramide<br>Flecainide<br>Mexiletine<br>Quinidine<br>Verapamil | Tablets<br>Tablets<br>Capsules<br>Tablets<br>Capsules<br>Tablets<br>Tablets | For the treatment of irregularities in the normal heart rhythm | Headache, nausea, flushing dizziness and skin rashes. Amiodarone and Flecainide may cause disturbances in thyroid, liver and lung function |
| Anticoagulants | Warfarin | Tablets | To reduce the clotting tendency of the blood | May interact with other medicines. Dosage must be carefully controlled to avoid bleeding tendency |
| Anti-platelet drugs | Aspirin<br>Ticlopidine<br>Clopidogrel | Tablets<br>Tablets<br>Tablets | To thin the blood | Stomach upset, nausea, skin rashes, diarrhoea |
| Beta-blockers | Acebutalol<br>Atenolol<br>Bispoprolol<br>Labetalol<br>Metoprolol<br>Nadolol<br>Oxprenolol<br>Pindolol<br>Propranolol<br>Timolol | Tablets or capsules<br>Tablets or syrup<br>Tablets<br>Tablets<br>Tablets<br>Tablets<br>Tablets<br>Tablets<br>Tablets or capsules<br>Tablets | For the treatment of angina and hypertension. Also used to prevent further heart attacks in those who are at risk | Fatigue, lethargy, cold hands and feet, dry eyes, nausea and skin rashes. Some drugs in this group may cause worsening of asthma or wheezing |
| Calcium antagonists | Amlopidine<br>Diltiazem<br>Felopidine<br>Nicardipine<br>Nifedipine<br>Verapamil | Tablets<br>Tablets or capsules<br>Tablets<br>Capsules<br>Tablets or capsules<br>Tablets | For the treatment of angina and hypertension | Flushing, headache, nausea, dizziness and ankle swelling |

| Class of drug | Generic name | Administration | Uses | Possible side-effects |
|---|---|---|---|---|
| Cholesterol-lowering drugs | | | | |
| *Statins* | Atorvastatin | Tablets | To reduce blood cholesterol | Headache, indigestion and occasionally myositis |
| | Cerivastatin | Tablets | | |
| | Fluvastatin | Capsules | | |
| | Pravastatin | Tablets | | |
| | Simvastatin | Tablets | | |
| *Bile Resins* | Cholestyramine | Sachets | | Flatulence, bloating, heartburn and constipation |
| | Colestipol | Sachets | | |
| *Fibrates* | Bezafibrate | Tablets | | Nausea, rashes and headache |
| | Fenofibrate | Capsules | | |
| | Gemfibrozil | Capsules | | |
| Diuretics | Bendrofluazide | Tablets | For the treatment of hypertension | Rash, stomach upset, gout |
| | Bumetanide | Tablets | | |
| | Frusemide | Tablets | | |
| | Spironolactone | Tablets | | |
| Nitrates | Glyceryl Trinitrate | Under the tongue, tablets, skin patches, ointment, aerosol or spray | For the treatment of angina | Flushing, headache and dizziness |
| | Isosorbide mononitrate | Tablets or capsules | | |
| | Isosorbide dinitrate | Tablets, capsules or aerosol | | |
| Potassium channel activators | Nicorandil | Tablets | For the prevention and treatment of angina | Flushing, headache, dizziness, indigestion |

# 6

# After the heart attack or heart surgery

Having a heart attack or heart surgery is an experience few people ever forget. Arriving in the coronary care unit or operating theatre with all the monitors, dials and flashing lights is frightening enough, but then the realisation that what is happening is potentially life-threatening begins to sink in, and all sorts of questions will come flooding into your mind. Am I going to die? How will the family cope without me? Will I be able to get back to work? In the days after the event, you are likely to feel alternately angry, frustrated or tearful. And when the time comes to go home, you will probably feel very apprehensive about leaving the safety of a modern hospital environment. All these are perfectly normal, healthy reactions to such a major life event.

Once you're back home, you're faced with a different set of difficulties as a loving family which is not very well informed, is lacking in confidence and feeling very apprehensive about its charge, suddenly surrounds you. When in doubt, your partner and family will naturally tend to err on the side of caution and be overprotective towards you, so that restrictions become the order of the day. While perfectly understandable, this may heighten your own feelings of anxiety and frustration. Odd aches and pains, particularly around the chest and arms, may make you feel more anxious than usual, although such symptoms are, in fact, extremely common and quite normal. Furthermore, depending upon how much information the hospital gave you before discharge, you may be feeling unsure about what activities are allowed and what should be avoided. The aim of this chapter is to answer some of the more common questions about physical and emotional rehabilitation in the first few weeks and months following a heart attack or heart surgery. *If you are worried about symptoms or are unclear about your medication, you should consult your own doctor without delay.*

## What physical symptoms should I expect during recovery?

After a heart attack you will feel tired and you may have a slight temperature, which will settle as the healing process progresses. The damaged area of heart muscle cannot be repaired, but scar tissue begins to form and this scarring is usually complete four to six weeks after the heart attack. During this time, odd twinges in the chest area are not uncommon, although prolonged episodes of pain should be reported to your doctor.

For those who have had surgery, pain in the chest is common and may last for a long time. During the operation the breastbone is split to gain access to the heart and then closed using wire sutures (stitches). The rate of healing varies, depending upon age and other factors. If leg veins were taken for grafting into the heart, the legs may also be painful and swollen for several weeks or even longer. Some hospitals use special stockings for all cardiac surgery patients once they start moving around. These will improve the circulation in the legs and reduce the risk of venous thromboses.

## What emotional symptoms should I expect during recovery?

It is quite common and perfectly normal to feel tearful and depressed for a period following a heart attack or surgery. This is a natural reaction to the anxiety and physical trauma you have lived through, and is usually temporary. Mood changes, particularly irritability and a short temper, are also common. These symptoms usually settle down after a month or two, when life begins to get back to a more familiar routine. A small proportion of patients experience more prolonged depressive symptoms and may benefit from anti-depressant drugs.

Sleepless nights worrying about the future and whether you will have another attack are also common and normal. These are best dealt with by talking them through with your doctor or the trained rehabilitation staff at your local hospital (see below).

Some patients (perhaps one to five in every 100) experience some memory loss after bypass surgery. This is usually temporary and improves over the first four to six months after the operation.

## Is joining a cardiac rehabilitation programme a good idea?

Four to six weeks after a heart attack or heart surgery, your hospital may invite you to join a cardiac rehabilitation ('rehab' for short) programme. This usually involves attending once or twice a week for between six and eight weeks or more. A rehabilitation programme has three main elements:

*Education*: This will be useful to help you understand the nature of the problem, the importance of risk factors and what steps you can take to avoid problems in the future.

*Exercise*: A graded exercise programme will increase your confidence and help you return to normal daily activities.

*Group support*: Being able to talk and share worries and anxieties with others who have similar problems, is very helpful. It can also be great fun! Many patients stay in touch with each other long after the rehabilitation programme has ended.

So, if the hospital is reasonably easy to get to, a structured rehabilitation programme is a great idea. However, if you have a very long and involved journey, the hassle of getting there may outweigh the benefits. If this is the case, home rehabilitation with occasional nurse supervision is a perfectly good and safe alternative for most patients.

## How soon can I get back to work?

To a large extent, of course, the answer to this question depends upon what sort of job you do. Assuming that you are not a lumberjack, you can expect to be back at work after two or three months following a heart attack or heart surgery. If your job is more physically demanding, you may need a longer period off work. In any event, it is a good idea to start gradually – perhaps by working part-time – for the first month or so.

## What about physical activity?

It is interesting to note how attitudes to physical activity after a heart attack have changed over the years. In the 1930s strict procedures limited the amount of movement during the period in hospital, and once discharged, patients must have felt very frustrated and helpless, as all forms of physical activity were limited for at least one year. Today, patients begin their rehabilitation while still in hospital and graded physical exercise is a key element in the rehabilitative process. Some post-coronary and post-bypass patients even go on to complete marathons, although this is obviously not for everyone!

For the first four to six weeks at home, normal activities of daily living, including comfortable walking, should be encouraged. At the end of that period – but not before – you may join a cardiac rehabilitation programme or start a graded walking programme at home. The reason for the six-week wait is because the scar from a heart attack takes about that length of time to become firm, and vigorous physical activity during that period may cause thinning of the scarred wall, resulting in an aneurysm (a balloon-like swelling in the wall of the heart). An aneurysm may produce a variety of symptoms, including disturbances in heart rhythm, or even heart failure, which will prolong your recovery period.

The first and most important thing to keep in mind about physical activity is that you should *start slowly*. There are no prizes for overdoing it, unless you think a return to the coronary care unit is a prize. If you are enrolled in a hospital cardiac rehabilitation programme, you will probably do stretching exercises and then a variety of aerobic activities (exercises which improve the functioning of the heart and circulation). If you are at home, a good starting point is an eight-week walking programme, in which both the distance and the speed of the walk are gradually increased. Later on, you may wish to engage in more vigorous activities such as swimming, tennis, cycling or badminton, all of which are beneficial to the heart. You should, however, avoid activities that have a large isometric component – for example, lifting heavy suitcases – because these may put a considerable strain on the heart. All these points are covered in detail in Action File 4, p.131.

If you have undergone bypass surgery, you may well experience discomfort around the neck, shoulders and back as you begin a walking programme. This is a natural consequence of the wound to the chest wall and will improve as the healing continues, so don't worry about it. You may also feel a little short of breath in the early stages, but again, this will gradually disappear as you become fitter and more active.

## Should I join a gym or health club?

Joining a local gym or health club is well worth considering, but not until you have completed a period of rehabilitation, either in a hospital programme or by following a walking programme at home. In practice, therefore, you should delay joining until three or four months after your heart attack or surgery.

Exercising in a club or gymnasium has obvious advantages. You can go along with a friend and make it a social occasion and you can exercise in any weather. Nowadays, many of the better-quality health clubs have trained physical instructors who will be able to advise you about clothing, footwear, the most appropriate types of exercise and how to monitor your progress. It is, of course, essential to let the club know that you have a heart condition and they will normally ask you to obtain a letter from your doctor confirming that it is OK for you to start exercising. (Incidentally, it is probably best to avoid saunas, steam cabinets and hot jacuzzis.)

## What about sex?

It is common – indeed, almost the norm – for patients to lose interest in sex after a heart attack or heart surgery. Many people are reluctant to discuss this with their doctor, and lack of guidance leads to anxiety and loss of interest. Fear of suffering angina or another heart attack during intercourse may be part of the problem, but sometimes apathy towards sex is just one symptom of a more generalised depression. As confidence returns – and this is where a graded exercise programme is so essential – the situation gradually corrects itself. The general advice is to wait three to four weeks after the attack, or until you can take a brisk walk or climb two flights of stairs without difficulty, before returning to normal sexual activity.

But is it likely that sex could bring on another heart attack? The sex act results in changes in pulse rate and blood pressure similar to those induced by exercise. However, compared with most forms of exercise, the amount of work done by the heart during sexual intercourse is quite modest. If you can take a brisk walk without difficulty, the demands of sex are likely to be well within your physical capacity. So the vast majority of post-coronary patients can safely engage in sexual activity, without any fear of undue strain on the heart.

If you experience angina during sex, you can take some anti-anginal medication – for example, nitroglycerin spray – before starting. If you have had heart surgery, you will need to find a comfortable position, one that places as little stress on your chest wall as possible. Some drugs prescribed for heart problems may reduce your sex drive and if you feel this is the case, have a word with your doctor.

## When can I start driving again?

You are usually not allowed by law to drive your car for one month after a heart attack or heart surgery, although you don't need to notify the Driver and Vehicle Licensing Agency (DVLA). However, there are special regulations for those who drive for a living, such as bus and taxi drivers. If you fall into this category you can obtain advice from your doctor or the DVLA (see Appendix 1, p.230).

If you have undergone surgery, when you do start driving again, you can expect to feel some discomfort around the chest, shoulders and arms as you move the steering wheel. This will improve as you become stronger and the chest wound continues to heal.

You should notify your insurance company if you have had a heart attack or heart surgery. If you have any difficulty in continuing with your insurance, the British Heart Foundation can supply a list of insurance companies who are happy to assist people with heart problems (see Appendix 1, p.227).

## Is it safe to travel?

For the first few months after a heart attack or surgery, it is probably best to avoid travelling abroad. After that time – and assuming you have made an uneventful recovery – you can probably travel wherever you want, within reason. Obviously, whitewater rafting along the Colorado River or strenuous mountaineering expeditions are probably best avoided! If you have any doubts, check with your doctor. You should also clarify the terms of your holiday insurance and make sure it includes cover for heart conditions. If you are taking medication, do make sure you have an adequate supply and keep it in your *hand luggage* (it won't be much use locked away in the hold of the aircraft or ship).

If you are flying, make sure you drink plenty of fluids, such as water and soft drinks, and avoid alcohol. On a long flight you may become dehydrated and alcohol will tend to exacerbate this, making the blood thicker and more liable to clot. It's also a good idea to stand up and stretch regularly, especially during a long journey. Sitting in one position for long periods can lead to sluggish circulation in the leg veins, which may occasionally result in a blood clot forming. Finally, remember what was said above about lifting heavy suitcases and bear in mind that in some airports you may have to walk quite a long distance before you get to the departure lounge. Give yourself plenty of time for this and rest on the way if you wish.

## Do I need to worry about the weather?

Avoid extremes of weather or temperature. It is best not to participate in outdoor activities when it is snowing or very cold. It is also wise to avoid very hot climates.

## Can I drink alcohol?

A small amount of alcohol, such as a glass of wine or sherry, is quite acceptable. However, you should avoid drinking strong spirits such as brandy and keep your overall alcohol consumption well within the recommended safe-drinking guidelines. Alcohol is discussed in more detail in Action File 6, p.175.

## What tablets will I have to take?

There are many types of medication used to treat heart problems (see Chapter 5). Some are used to treat hypertension, angina or heart failure, and others to lower cholesterol levels or to control abnormal heart rhythms. What you are prescribed, therefore, will depend upon whether you have any of these problems. You may well require a combination of drugs, which will probably include aspirin, beta-blockers and ACE inhibitors, because they have been shown in scientific studies to reduce the risk of further heart attacks.

## What else can I do to reduce my risk of further heart problems?

Lots! Some patients feel that having had a heart attack or heart surgery the damage is already done, and that it's too late to modify lifestyle factors such as smoking, physical activity and diet. Nothing could be further from the truth. By paying attention to your cholesterol levels, taking proper exercise, keeping your weight and blood pressure under control and making modest changes in your diet, you really can lower your risks and avoid further problems. In fact, many patients become fitter and healthier after a heart attack than they were before. (See Part II, p.91 – where the counter-attack begins!)

# 7

# Hormones and the heart

From the onset of menstruation at puberty, through pregnancy and lactation in early adult life, to the menopause in later life, a woman's hormones play a central role in her physical, emotional and sexual well-being. But using hormonal supplements has implications which extend well beyond considerations of contraception, fertility and the relief of menopausal symptoms. It is quite clear that taking oestrogens and progestogens (the female sex hormones) can have an important effect on the risk for heart attack and other circulatory problems.

Sex hormones are used in two main forms: oral contraceptives (OCs) and hormone replacement therapy (HRT). These and related issues are described here under the following headings:

- The oral contraceptive pill
- The menopause and heart disease
- HRT and CHD risk

## The oral contraceptive pill

The oral contraceptive pill contains a combination of synthetic oestrogen and progestogen in varying proportions. One of the difficulties in studying the effects of the Pill is that these two ingredients have different – in fact, opposite – effects. In general, oestrogens tend to increase HDL-C ('good' cholesterol) whilst lowering LDL-C ('bad' cholesterol), the effect being to *reduce* the risk of heart disease. Conversely, progestogens tend to increase LDL-C and reduce HDL-C, thus tending to *increase* the risk of heart attack. Hence the net effect of any Pill preparation depends to a great extent upon the relative amounts of oestrogen and progestogen in the formulation being used.

Apart from the risk of heart attack, there is also the worry about venous thrombosis. Soon after the Pill became available in 1960, multiple cases of venous thrombosis were reported. It is now clear that the 'early generation' of high-dose oestrogen and progestogen preparations increased the tendency to form blood clots, especially in those who smoked. Doses of both oestrogen and progestogen have been reduced a great deal in recent years, so that 'second' and 'third' generation oral contraceptives are now very much safer. So what does the current evidence say about the risk of blood clots and heart attacks with use of the contraceptive pill?

## Venous thrombosis

The risk of venous thrombosis (blood clots in the legs) in those taking modern 'low-dose' Pill formulations is very small. In fact, the risk of a venous thrombosis in a normal pregnancy is two to four times higher than that associated with the Pill. *However, the combination of smoking and the Pill increases the risk dramatically.*

There is also an increased risk of venous thrombosis in women who have a genetic blood disorder called Factor V Leiden, which affects around five per cent of Caucasians (although it is virtually absent in Africans and Asians). Screening for Factor V Leiden is recommended for all women who have a history of venous thrombosis, since they form a particularly high risk group.

## Heart attack

With respect to heart disease, in the absence of cigarette smoking, there is no real evidence that use of the modern low-dose contraceptive pill significantly increases heart attack risk. However, women who both smoke and use the Pill – particularly women over 35 – increase their risk of a heart attack at least five times compared with non-smoking non-users. Thus it is smoking, and not the pill, that constitutes the greater cardiovascular risk. There is also a slightly increased risk of a heart attack in Pill-users who are hypertensive, compared with Pill-users with normal blood pressure. There is, incidentally, no evidence to suggest an increased risk of heart disease among past users of the Pill – even with prolonged use.

*Summary*: The excess risk of venous thrombosis and heart attack in women who use the Pill, is very small and largely confined to smokers, particularly those over 35 years old. There is no increase in risk for past users of the Pill.

# The menopause and heart disease

## What is the menopause?

The menopause – also called the 'change of life' – usually occurs around the age of 50 and is said to have begun when a woman has not had a period for a year. Of course, many women experience menopausal symptoms and irregular periods for several years before the menopause itself. This is called the 'climacteric' and represents the gradual decline in the normal function of the ovaries.

Over the last century, female life expectancy has steadily increased, while the average age of the menopause (51.4 years) has not changed in over 200 years. Today, the average woman can expect to spend about one-third of her life in the postmenopausal state and, consequently, doctors are seeing the effects of menopause-associated hormonal changes much more frequently. Research into the menopause is relatively recent. A hundred years ago, when life expectancy was much shorter than it is today, women did not live very long after the menopause and so little was known about it.

## Why does it occur?

The menopause occurs because the ovaries lose their ability to perform the function of ovulation (producing an egg) each month. At the same time, they are no longer able to produce the two main female sex hormones, oestrogen and progestogen. It is the fall in the blood levels of these hormones which may give rise to the symptoms of menopause.

## What are the symptoms?

Eventually, nearly every woman learns about the symptoms of menopause – the gradual decline in regular menstruation and, for many women, hot flushes and mood changes. How women experience the menopausal transition depends on a host of factors, including heredity, medical history, diet, exercise, expectations and cultural background. Many women sail through it without experiencing any troublesome symptoms whatever.

But of greater importance than the more obvious symptoms are the silent effects of the menopause on the body, ranging from loss of calcium in the bones to effects on the cardiovascular system, including changes in blood cholesterol levels and other risk factors. Nowadays, the effects of the menopause on the heart and blood vessels are of great interest, both for doctors and women themselves, because of the widespread view that some of the unwanted consequences can be reversed through hormone replacement therapy (HRT).

## Heart disease and the menopause 'myth'

So what effect does reaching the menopause have on your risk of getting heart disease? Because death rates from heart disease in women under 50 are low, the assumption has always been that prior to the menopause women are protected against heart disease by their hormones, particularly oestrogens. As ovarian function falters around the menopause, or so the argument goes, oestrogen levels fall and, as a direct consequence, death rates from heart disease in women suddenly rise (see Figure 19a).

*Figure 19* CHD and the menopause 'myth'

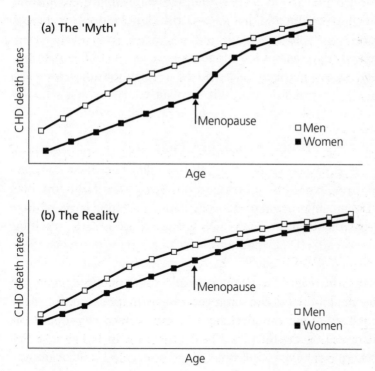

However, while this account of events is the one promoted by women's magazines, the media and (for obvious reasons), the pharmaceutical industry, *it is wrong.*

There *is* no sudden increase in heart disease rates after the menopause. On the contrary, the rate of increase in women aged 30–34 through to 60–64 years is almost the same (see Figure 19b). The number of women with heart attacks increases after the age of 50, but this is due to the continuing effect of age, not the menopause. And the reason why the death rates in women and men are similar in older age groups is not because rates increase in women, but because they fall slightly in men.

# HRT and CHD risk

But even if there is no sudden increase in death rates after the menopause, does taking HRT reduce the risks of heart disease in those who take it? After all, many doctors now recommend HRT for the prevention of heart disease and osteoporosis (loss of bone mineral), as well as for the relief of menopausal symptoms. In Britain about one quarter of women aged 50–64 – some 1.3 million – take HRT and presumably many, if not most, of these women have been told that a lower risk of heart disease is one of the benefits.

Given the wide coverage of the supposed benefits of HRT in the popular press and media, you may be surprised to learn that the answer to the question is not straightforward. To explain why, let's first see *why* HRT should reduce risk and then see *whether* it actually does so.

## Why should HRT reduce the risk of CHD?

There are good reasons to suggest that HRT should be beneficial in terms of heart health. As with the oral contraceptive pill, most HRT formulations consist of a combination of oestrogen and progestogen. As we saw earlier, oestrogen tends to increase HDL-C and reduce LDL-C, resulting in a lower risk of CHD. In addition, oestrogen improves blood flow through the arteries, and reduces the tendency of the blood to clot – further reducing the risk of heart attack. While it is theoretically true that progestogens tend to have the opposite effect, in practice the small amounts contained in most modern HRT preparations do not appear to have any unwanted effects. (Incidentally, the reason why a progestogen is added is because oestrogen used alone may increase the risk of uterine cancer, i.e. cancer of the womb. The addition of a progestogen almost eliminates this risk).

## Does HRT reduce the risk of heart attack?

So does the predicted reduction in the risk of heart attack for women taking HRT actually happen in practice?

Many studies have indeed demonstrated a reduction in CHD risk among HRT-users compared with non-users. Moreover, the size of the potential benefit – up to 50 per cent reduction in risk for women using hormones – is impressive. The problem is that many of these studies were flawed and their conclusions cannot be regarded as entirely reliable. In some, for example, women who became unwell while taking HRT withdrew from the group, leaving only the healthier women behind. In others it was found that the women taking HRT had lower levels of CHD risk factors than the non-users *before* starting treatment. Because the rates of heart attack are likely to be much lower in these healthy subjects, it *looked* as though HRT was protecting them, when in fact they did better simply because they were healthier to start with (known as 'healthy user bias'). It is, therefore, quite possible that the apparent benefits of HRT with respect to heart disease are either exaggerated or entirely absent.

In order to resolve the issue of whether HRT really is beneficial in terms of heart disease prevention after the menopause, we need *randomised trials*. Several such trials in healthy women are already underway, but it is likely to be some years before the full results are available. At the time of writing, preliminary results from a large American study, The Women's Health Initiative, seem to suggest that HRT may not reduce the risk of cardiovascular disease, but instead may even increase it! Now, these are very early results and the eventual conclusion of the trial may be quite different. However, it does suggest that the reported benefits from previous, less rigorous studies may have been wildly optimistic.

*Summary*: The apparent benefit of HRT in terms of protection against cardiovascular disease observed in earlier studies could be due to the fact that women taking HRT tended to be healthier to begin with. The effect of this healthy user bias can be substantial and could easily account for the 40–50 per cent reduction in heart disease risk which is often attributed to HRT. When these things are taken into account, along with preliminary results from randomised trials, we have to conclude that the case for HRT – at least in terms of CVD – has yet to be made.

## What about women who already have heart disease?

A preliminary answer to this question has come from the HERS (Heart and Oestrogen/Progestogen Replacement Study) involving 2763 women with established heart disease. Women were divided into two groups: those taking HRT and those taking a placebo pill. At the end of four years, there was no overall difference in heart attack rates between the two groups. In other words, HRT did not benefit women who already had evidence of heart disease.

## What are the benefits of HRT?

Although the case has yet to be made in terms of the benefits of HRT for heart disease, there are other reasons why a doctor may decide to prescribe HRT in any individual case:

- Menopausal symptoms such as flushing and night sweats usually respond promptly to treatment.
- HRT can improve bone density and reduce the risk of hip fracture by 30 per cent and spinal fracture by 50 per cent. However, if used for the prevention of osteoporosis and bone fracture, HRT must be used indefinitely. In one study, 10 years after HRT had been stopped, bone density and fracture risk were similar in women who had used oestrogen replacement and those who had not.
- There is also some early research evidence to suggest that HRT users may have a lower risk of Alzheimer's disease (dementia) and cancer of the bowel.
- HRT is easy to take and is available in different forms to suit individual preferences, for example, tablets, skin patches, implants under the skin or as a gel applied to the skin each day.

## What are the risks of HRT?

There are three main risks associated with oestrogen replacement or HRT:

- Breast cancer
- Venous thrombosis
- Uterine cancer (cancer of the womb)

The risk of breast cancer is real and is related to the length of time HRT is taken. For the first four or five years the risk is minimal – good news if you are taking it during the peri-menopause ('climacteric'). But taking HRT for more than five years increases the risk of breast cancer by 30 per cent. This does not mean that women should automatically stop taking HRT after five years, but they should attend for regular breast screening and examine their breasts for lumps regularly. Women with a history of breast cancer, or who have close relatives with the disease, should see a specialist before starting on HRT. Incidentally, the small risk of breast cancer disappears entirely within five years of stopping HRT medication, even after a long period of use.

Hormone replacement may also increase the risk of venous thrombosis, although in practice this excess risk is actually quite small – about one in every 5000 users per year. Women with a previous episode of thrombosis, or with close relatives who have had a thrombosis, need special blood tests before starting HRT. With regard to uterine cancer, the risk (as indicated earlier) is largely removed by the addition of a progestogen.

## The $64,000 question – who should take HRT?

The potential risks and benefits of taking HRT are summarised below.

*Table 5*  HRT – benefits and risks

---

*Benefits*
Reduced risk of heart disease (unproven)
Reduced menopausal symptoms
Reduced risk of osteoporosis & bone fracture
Reduced risk of Alzheimer's disease
Reduced risk of bowel cancer

*Risks*
Increased risk of breast cancer
Increased risk of venous thrombosis
Increased risk of uterine cancer

---

If we assume that the benefits of HRT in terms of heart disease are unproven – at least for the moment – then the main arguments for taking it are for the relief of menopausal symptoms such as night sweats, hot flushes, mood swings and fatigue, and for the prevention and treatment of osteoporosis (NB: The evidence for protection against bowel cancer and Alzheimer's is very preliminary).

The use of HRT in the short term to reduce menopausal symptoms is unlikely to be a problem. However, longer-term use of HRT for the prevention or treatment of bone disease in an otherwise healthy woman is much more of a dilemma, and the risks and benefits must be carefully weighed. For example, a woman with normal bone density and a family history of breast cancer should *not* take HRT in the long term. On the other hand, a woman with low bone density – particularly if she has already suffered bone fractures – and who has an average risk of breast cancer, may be a good candidate for HRT. The dilemma, of course, is that to get the benefit of HRT in terms of osteoporosis, it has to be taken indefinitely, and yet the longer treatment continues, the greater the risk of breast cancer.

It's all a question of balancing the risks against the benefits in your own case. This can only be done after careful discussion with your family doctor. In the end, it just comes down to where you would prefer to put your risks. And remember, you can always change your mind!

*Summary*: Our culture has gone from ignoring the menopause to medicalising it. Western medicine now sees this normal life transition as an oestrogen-deficiency disease, brought on by 'ovarian failure'. Many doctors are enthusiastic advocates of HRT, and yet many women manage perfectly well without it. Moreover, of the women who start, half stop within a year.

The idea of taking an anti-ageing pill in the form of HRT is clearly attractive to many women, and one that is heavily promoted by the media and pharmaceutical companies. But in fact HRT is unlikely to be the solution to healthy ageing in women. The large international variations in chronic disease strongly suggest that many conditions such as heart and bone disease are potentially preventable, and are not due to the menopause *per se*. For example, Japanese women have naturally *low* levels of oestrogen and yet they have the lowest rates for coronary disease, a low level of menopausal symptoms and the greatest longevity. The use of HRT should not divert attention away from other, more important determinants of women's heart health.

# PART II

## Action File 1
# Smoking – how to stop and stay stopped

---

Cigarette-smoking remains the leading preventable cause of heart disease in women. Even if you only smoke one to four cigarettes per day, your risk of both fatal and non-fatal heart attack is two and a half times greater than that of non-smoking women. Those who already have heart problems but who continue to smoke are at especially high risk. Nicotine – the active drug in tobacco – is highly addictive, which is why many people find it difficult to stop. Difficult maybe, but by no means impossible. Success requires careful planning and preparation, combined with great personal commitment. Family and friends can provide support and there are also professional organisations that can give advice and encouragement. Giving up smoking is the most important single contribution you can make to your future health and well-being. Reading through this section will help you to set the date to quit – and achieve your goal!

---

## Background

The American writer Mark Twain once said, 'Quitting smoking is easy. I've done it a thousand times.' Perhaps you have tried to stop too – most smokers have at one time or another. But why do people find it so difficult?

The answer is that nicotine, the active drug found in tobacco, is highly addictive and, as with any addiction, breaking the habit can be extraordinarily difficult. Smoking produces both a physical and a psychological dependence. The physical dependence which cigarettes engender is very real – although smokers develop a tolerance to nicotine, withdrawal symptoms *do* occur when it is withheld. The psychological dependence is equally real – as any regular smoker will tell you.

### Smoking – the risks

Although giving up the habit is difficult, the incentives for doing so are overwhelming. Indeed, if you do only one thing as a result of reading this book, you should stop smoking. Everyone knows about the various risks – rehearsing the details again here is pointless. But the salient facts are:

- Cigarette smoking is a major risk factor for the development of heart disease in women and also for many other serious illnesses, including cancer and lung disease.
- Smoking is a more potent risk factor for heart attacks in women, than in men.
- Women who smoke as few as one to four cigarettes per day have two and a half times the risk of both fatal and non-fatal heart attack compared with non-smoking women.
- Among women who had their first heart attack before the age of 50, over 60 per cent of cases can be attributed to cigarette smoking.
- Smoking remains the leading preventable cause of heart disease in women, with more than 50 per cent of heart attacks in middle-aged women attributable to tobacco.
- Smoking and the oral contraceptive pill are a particularly dangerous combination.
- There is a clear relationship between smoking and complications during pregnancy.

*Smoking for those who already have a history of heart problems is – and there is no other way to say it – lethal.*

You may also be interested to know that in Caucasian women smoking is related to wrinkling of the skin which can sometimes be an effective motivator to give up!

## What's in tobacco smoke and what makes it so dangerous?

Cigarettes contain more than 4000 chemical compounds and at least 400 poisonous substances. The substances most damaging to health are tar (associated with lung cancer), carbon monoxide and nicotine (associated with heart disease and stroke) and other harmful particles and gases (associated with chronic lung disease).

When tobacco smoke is inhaled, nicotine and other harmful substances are carried deep into the lungs, where they are quickly absorbed into the bloodstream and carried to the heart, brain and liver. Nicotine produces pleasurable feelings that make you want to smoke more, but also acts as a depressant by interfering with the flow of information between nerve cells. Nicotine is as addictive as cocaine and heroin and, as mentioned above, the body becomes both physically and psychologically dependent upon it. Studies show that smokers have to overcome both of these dependencies to be successful at giving up.

Mainstream smoke is the smoke inhaled directly by the smoker, while 'side stream' smoke is the smoke that comes off the tip of the cigarette in between puffs. Paradoxically, the side stream smoke carries a greater concentration of harmful substances than directly inhaled smoke and is, therefore, a greater health risk. The smoker inhales both mainstream and side stream smoke, while the non-smoker (passive smoker) inhales the more dangerous side stream smoke, as well as the smoke breathed out by the person with the cigarette.

## Is passive smoking dangerous?

Yes. Evidence shows that women exposed to side stream smoke – either at home or in the workplace – have nearly double the risk of heart disease than women who are not exposed. Passive smoking like this is particularly dangerous for those who already have heart problems. Moreover, babies and young children raised in a household where there is smoking, have more ear infections, colds, bronchitis and other lung problems than children from non-smoking families. So if you smoke, it is not only your own health that will suffer, but also the health of all those around you. This is why non-smokers have good reason to be concerned about inhaling other people's smoke.

## What about smoking during pregnancy

There is compelling evidence that cigarette-smoking during pregnancy can have a damaging effect upon the developing child. Babies of mothers who smoke:

- Are more likely to be born prematurely.
- Have a birth weight on average 200g (7oz) less then those born to non-smokers.
- Have organs that are smaller on average than babies born to non-smokers. This is especially true in the case of the lungs of the newborn baby which do not function as well as the lungs of babies born to non-smoking mothers.
- Are twice as likely to die from cot death.
- Are more likely to become smokers themselves.

Pregnant women who smoke also increase their risk of early miscarriage. In the later stages of pregnancy, there is a greater risk that the placenta will come away from the womb before the baby is born – known as placental abruption. This may, in turn, cause the baby to be born prematurely, starved of oxygen or even stillborn.

## Is it better to smoke low tar cigarettes?

Smoking a low-tar cigarette does not reduce the risk of developing heart disease or other forms of chronic lung disease. Many smokers who switch to low-tar brands inhale more deeply, take more puffs per cigarette and smoke more cigarettes than before. Low-tar cigarettes are, however, probably less dangerous than high-tar cigarettes with respect to lung cancer. This is because the concentration of cancer-causing agents in a low-tar cigarette is significantly lower than in a high-tar cigarette. Nevertheless, even smoking low-tar brands carries a significantly increased risk of cancer when compared with not smoking at all.

The only safe cigarette is the one that hasn't been smoked.

# Action plan

If you are a smoker, the first thing you have to do is decide whether you really want to stop. This – to state the obvious – is a decision that only you can make. Your partner, family and friends may want you to stop, but the commitment must come from you.

Doctors have tried to understand why and how some people stop smoking, while others never manage to do so. They have developed different ideas or 'models' which describe the various stages most smokers go through when trying to give up. One of these is called the *Stages of Change Model* which consists of the following stages:

**Pre-Contemplation:** When the smoker is not thinking seriously about stopping at the moment.

**Contemplation:** When the smoker is actively thinking about stopping, but is still not ready to make a determined attempt. Excuses such as 'There's a lot going on, and trying to stop smoking as well is just too much for me at the moment' are common at this stage.

**Preparation:** When the smoker has decided to stop in the near future and usually has a date in mind – for example, a New Year's resolution.

**Action:** The initial six-month period when the smoker is actively stopping.

**Maintenance:** The period between six months and five years when the ex-smoker is aware of the danger of relapse and takes active steps to avoid it.

What stage are you at in this model? Psychologically, you need to get yourself into the preparation stage so that you can set a date and make a plan.

It is also useful to get a sense of how strongly you are addicted to nicotine. Take a minute or two to complete the following questionnaire, which measures your physical dependency on the nicotine in cigarettes. If you find that your level of addiction is high, you may benefit from some form of nicotine replacement therapy earlier rather than later in your stop-smoking plan.

---

### NICOTINE DEPENDENCE QUESTIONNAIRE

**To calculate your nicotine addiction score, simply add up the points (in brackets) allocated to each question according to your response.**

1.  How many cigarettes a day do you smoke?
    0–15 [0]    16–25 [1]    25+ [3]

2.  What is the nicotine yield per cigarette of your usual brand?
    0.3–0.8g [0]    0.9–1.5g [1]    1.6–2.2g [2]

3.  Do you inhale?
    Never [0]    Sometimes [1]    Always [2]

4.  Do you smoke more during the morning than during the rest of the day?
    No [0]    Yes [1]

5.  How soon after you wake up do you smoke your first cigarette?
    More than 30 mins [0]    Less than 30 mins [1]

6.  Of all the cigarettes you smoke during the day, which would you most hate to give up?
    The first of the day [1]    All other answers [0]

7.  Do you find it difficult not to smoke in places where smoking is prohibited (eg. cinema, library, on an aeroplane etc)?
    No [0]    Yes [1]

8.  Would you smoke even if you were so ill that you had to stay in bed most of the day?
    No [0]    Yes [1]

Score _____

**Interpretation**
*Score    Level of Nicotine Dependence*
0–3    Low
4–7    Moderate
8–11    High

## Stopping 1: Set the date

Let's assume you have decided to stop; what next? The first and most important step is to name the day – decide *when* you intend to stop or begin to cut down. Choose a day within the next month as your stopping day. This should be long enough to give yourself some time to adjust to the idea and prepare, but not too far distant for you to find new reasons to change your mind! When you have set the date, here are some things you can do to prepare:

- Mark the date on the calendar.
- Tell family, friends and work colleagues.
- Decide on a plan. Will you join a stop-smoking class or use nicotine replacement therapy? Is there a friend who has managed to stop and who is prepared to offer support?
- Plan other health strategies – for example, join a health club, take more exercise and pay more attention to your diet. Buy yourself some new exercise wear and sports trainers.
- Start thinking of yourself as a non-smoker; practise saying, 'No thanks, I don't smoke.'

There is no right way to stop smoking. Many people – perhaps most – decide to go 'cold turkey', and just stop completely. Others prefer to reduce their dependence on nicotine slowly, by gradually reducing the consumption of cigarettes – a process called 'nicotine fading'. To do this:

- Switch to a lower-nicotine level cigarette.
- Gradually reduce the number of cigarettes you're smoking.
- Put the cigarette out earlier than normal.
- Try to inhale less deeply.

By planning this over a period of a few weeks, you can get your consumption down to, say, 10 cigarettes per day, at which point you can decide to stop completely.

Whether you decide to stop completely all at once, or use the 'nicotine fading' approach, it's important not to underestimate the difficulty of what you're trying to achieve. There is no magic formula that's going to make you into a non-smoker overnight. Success depends upon proper preparation, combined with iron determination.

## Stopping 2: The big day

On the big day, get rid of all smoking materials – cigarette packets, lighters and matches, ashtrays, etc. Have your clothes cleaned or buy some new outfits. Then practice the 'Four As': **Avoid**, **Alter**, **Alternatives** and **Activities**.

**Avoid**: Try to avoid people and places where you are likely to smoke.

**Alter**: Alter parts of your daily routine such as taking a different route to work, going to the health-club or gym at a time when you may be tempted to smoke. Spend less time on activities such as watching TV or reading, where you may be tempted to start smoking again. Drink lots of water and fruit juices instead of coffee or alcohol.

**Alternatives**: Start using oral substitutes such as sugarless chewing gum, raw vegetables and fruit such as carrot sticks, slices of apple or celery. If you have decided to use nicotine replacement (patches, gum or spray etc), you should start now.

**Activities**: Being physically active and finding a new hobby will help to distract you from any withdrawal symptoms and the urge to smoke. The key thing is not to give yourself the time to think about whether you are missing the cigarettes.

## Dealing with withdrawal

When smokers cut back or stop altogether, the lack of nicotine leads to a well recognised withdrawal syndrome, which includes depression, irritability, difficulty in concentrating, restlessness, insomnia, headache, tiredness and increased appetite. If your dependence on nicotine is high then you should assume that your withdrawal symptoms may be quite severe and be prepared.

Some tips for dealing with some of the more common withdrawal symptoms are as follows:

- **Craving:** More than 90 per cent of smokers will experience cigarette cravings during withdrawal. If you have been a heavy smoker, these will usually last for about three weeks, gradually easing off. One way to help overcome this problem is to find some way to distract yourself each time you feel the craving. Go to the toilet, make some coffee, hang a picture, play the piano – do anything to distract yourself. If there are certain parts of your routine which you invariably associate with smoking a cigarette, such as reading the paper, then don't read it. If you normally have a cigarette at the end of a meal, have a mint and brush your teeth instead. If you are eating out, eat in the No Smoking part of the restaurant. Nicotine substitutes (see overleaf) can be a great help in dealing with cigarette cravings.

- **Irritability, anxiety and loss of concentration:** Most of these can be attributed to the upheaval of breaking a long-established habit as well as trying to adjust to the physical problems. There is no easy answer to this, and it may take two to three months to adjust. The support of those around you, both at work and at home, can be critical during this period.
- **Worsening cough:** As your body tries to rid itself of all the filth caused by cigarette-smoking, you may experience a temporary worsening of your smoker's cough. This will disappear after a few weeks or so.
- **Feeling light-headed or dizzy:** This tends to be a short-lived symptom, usually lasting for only 7–10 days. Other minor symptoms include nausea, constipation or diarrhoea and occasional headaches. Again, these should disappear after a couple of weeks.

## Nicotine substitutes

The nicotine patch, gum and nasal spray are medicines which provide nicotine, without all the other harmful components of tobacco. It is the highly addictive nature of nicotine which makes it so hard to quit, which is where replacement therapy like this can help. Nicotine substitutes have been well researched and tests have shown that, if used correctly, they can double your chances of success.

Nicotine replacement products are generally safer than cigarettes, *but if you have or have had a heart problem, you must check with your doctor or pharmacist before starting to use them.* In particular, you must stop smoking completely while you are using it. The four main forms of nicotine replacement therapy available at the moment are:

- gum (e.g. Nicorette)
- patches (e.g. Nicorette, Nicotinell)
- nasal spray (e.g. Nicorette)
- inhalator (e.g. Nicorette)

For all these products, it is essential to read the manufacturer's instructions for correct use. If you are unsure, ask your pharmacist or doctor for advice.

The patch provides a continual supply of nicotine at a low dose while you are wearing it, so it is not easy to respond quickly to a craving or a stressful moment. The nasal spray, gum and inhalator deliver a high dose of nicotine rapidly, so you can take a 'quick fix' when you need it.

When choosing which type of replacement therapy to use, you should think about which method will best suit your lifestyle and smoking pattern. If you tend to smoke steadily throughout the day, for example, the patch may be your best option. If, on the other hand, you smoke mainly in response to stressful events or situations, the gum, spray or inhalator may be preferable. The inhalator is particularly helpful if you miss the 'hand to mouth' action of smoking a cigarette.

Side-effects of nicotine replacement include nausea, headache, indigestion, dizziness and palpitations, but these tend to improve with use. If you experience problems with one form of nicotine substitute, it's worth swapping and trying one or two of the others.

## Other drugs

A new antidepressant drug called Buproprion (Zyban) appears to be effective in helping smokers to quit. The logic behind this discovery is that in some smokers, nicotine acts as an antidepressant; when they eventually decide to quit, they become depressed. Because Buproprion helps to offset the depression which otherwise occurs, ex-smokers are less likely to start again. It also appears to prevent some of the weight gain associated with stopping smoking (see p.103). Buproprion is now generally available in the UK on prescription, although it should be used with caution in patients with known heart problems. Other anti-depressant drugs such as Doxepin (Sinequan) and Nortripyline (Allegron) may also be helpful, although they may sometimes have unpleasant side-effects.

## Other ways to stop smoking

There are lots of other aids to quitting smoking, which are easily available through mail order, newsagents, health shops, pharmacies and the Internet. Options include scented inhalers, dummy cigarettes, tobacco-flavoured chewing gum, herbal cigarettes and filters. There is little or no scientific evidence to say how effective these remedies are, but you should be wary of claims for high success rates. Filters, in particular, are not usually effective, since studies show that smokers who use them actually smoke more.

Alternative therapies can sometimes be useful. Acupuncture has been used to help people quit smoking, although there is very little evidence to support the claims made for its effectiveness, and hypnosis may also be helpful in some cases. If you *do* decide to opt for alternative therapies, however, it is important to find a registered practitioner.

Support groups can be very useful for some people. They are usually run over a period of weeks and take you step-by-step through the various stages of stopping. There are also specialist stop smoking clinics, providing nicotine replacement products, which may improve your chances of stopping three- or four-fold.

> *Whichever method you choose to stop smoking, it is essential to think it through carefully in advance and make sure you have a clear plan of action.*

If you would like further information about support groups, clinics or smoking cessation products, then QUITLINE® can help. This is a free telephone helpline for people who want to stop smoking. QUITLINE® has trained counsellors who can provide support and encouragement while you are trying to stop and who can answer any questions you may have about specific smoking cessation products and programmes (See Appendix 1, p.232).

## Stopping 3: Staying stopped

Once you have managed to negotiate the first six months or so without a cigarette, you may think you are over the worst and that it's time to relax. Not so! There are still going to be times when the urge to start smoking again will be difficult to resist and your greatest enemy at this stage is *complacency*. Again, the important point here is to think ahead, anticipate the problems well in advance and prepare for them.

To get through the times of temptation, it is useful to:

- Rehearse in your mind all the reasons why you chose to quit in the first place.
- Remind yourself that there is no such thing as *just one cigarette*. Don't delude yourself that it will only be one – or even one puff.
- Do something. If you find yourself in a situation where the temptation arises, get yourself out of there!

It is also useful to set aside all the money you would normally spend on cigarettes – you will be pleasantly surprised at how quickly it mounts up. Plan to treat yourself to something you have wanted for a long time (not a new cigarette lighter!). Take pride in your improving health and appearance. You must constantly reinforce success in your own mind – don't anticipate failure.

But what if you do succumb and have that cigarette? The key now is not to allow a *slip* to become a *relapse*. Don't use the slip as an excuse to start smoking again. Use it as an opportunity to understand what went wrong, to learn and to renew your commitment – then move on.

## How soon will I benefit from stopping?

The benefits of stopping smoking begin immediately and apply to women of all ages. The main ones are as follows:

- Within 24 hours of stopping your risk of a heart attack begins to decrease.
- One to three months after stopping, morning cough and sinus congestion decrease, lung function is up by 30 per cent and shortness of breath decreases.
- Within one year of stopping, your risk of heart disease will be reduced by about a half and within 15 years it will be the same as if you had never smoked.
- Within five to 15 years of stopping, your risk of stroke will be the same as those who have never smoked.
- Women who quit between the age of 35 to 39 add an average of five years to their lives. Even those who stop between the ages of 65 to 69, increase their life expectancy by one year.

## Will I gain weight?

One of the excuses for not giving up smoking, particularly among women, is that it's a short cut to gaining weight. Many women who return to smoking after having stopped, do so with the deliberate intention of controlling their weight. So what are the facts?

Studies show that about 80 per cent of successful quitters gain weight – on average around 1.8Kg (4–6lb), although a small percentage may gain considerably more than this. Women appear to be more likely to suffer higher weight gains after smoking cessation, although the reasons for this are not clear. Part of the explanation may be due to dietary changes, in particular increased consumption of sweets and carbohydrates. However, it may also be that stopping smoking decreases the resting metabolic rate (p.165).

However, the point about this modest weight gain is that it *does not* appear to increase the risk of heart disease. So in terms of the risk of heart disease, stopping smoking – even if this is followed by some weight gain – is probably the most important single step you can take (leaving aside all the other appalling health consequences of continuing to smoke).

But, I hear you say, I still don't like the idea of putting on those extra pounds. Is there anything I can do to prevent this? The answer is that close attention to your diet and physical activity patterns will certainly help, although their impact is usually modest. There is evidence that the use of nicotine substitutes can offset the weight gain. Buproprion may help you to stop smoking whilst reducing the amount of weight gained.

## What if I really can't stop?

Obviously nothing is going to make smoking safe, and anything short of stopping completely is a compromise. However, it is a compromise that you may wish to accept. If this is the case, there are still some steps you can take to limit the harm from cigarettes.

- Choose low-tar cigarettes.
- Don't smoke your cigarettes all the way down; you get most of the tar and nicotine from the last few drags. If you smoke half you will only get about 40 per cent of the total tar and nicotine.
- Take fewer drags on each cigarette.
- Try not to inhale as much smoke.
- Try to smoke fewer cigarettes each day. Perhaps you might like to consider not smoking at home, or only smoking at set times.

To end this important section, here is your Stop Smoking checklist:

---

### A CHECKLIST FOR STOPPING SMOKING

✓ Set the date and tell your partner, family and friends

✓ Make a plan well in advance – e.g. consider smoking cessation classes

✓ Plan other health strategies, such as taking exercise and improving your diet

✓ On the day, remember the 4 As – Avoid, Alter, Alternatives and Activities

✓ Use nicotine substitutes appropriately

✓ Don't be too concerned about weight gain

✓ Stay stopped – don't be complacent! Try to anticipate difficulties and plan for them well in advance. Remember the health benefits.

---

# Action File 2

# Lowering your cholesterol level

Blood cholesterol and other lipids are major risk factors for heart disease. Keeping your cholesterol at a healthy level is, therefore, very important, all the more so if you already have a history of heart disease. Fortunately, it's not too difficult to lower your blood cholesterol. By following a cholesterol-lowering diet (low in saturated fat but rich in fresh fruit, fish and vegetables), keeping your alcohol intake within sensible limits, maintaining a healthy weight and taking regular exercise, you *can* get your cholesterol down – and keep it there! Modern drugs can also help – but must always be combined with lifestyle measures.

## Background

Cholesterol is a soft, waxy substance found among the lipids (fats) in the bloodstream and in all the cells of the body, especially those of the brain, spinal cord and nerves. It is also required for the manufacture of hormones, including cortisone and the sex hormones. In short, you could not live without it. The problem is that when levels of cholesterol in the blood are too high – a condition called *hypercholesterolaemia* – the formation of arterial plaque is accelerated and the risk of heart disease rises.

### Types of cholesterol

Cholesterol and other lipids cannot dissolve in the blood and have to be transported to and from the cells by special carriers called lipoproteins. There are several different forms of cholesterol in the blood, depending upon which lipoprotein carrier is being used. The two main carrier forms are low-density lipoprotein cholesterol (LDL-C) and high-density lipoprotein cholesterol (HDL-C), with a small amount of cholesterol carried by other lipoproteins (see Figure 20).

LDL-C usually carries about 70 per cent of the choles-terol in the blood. When blood levels of LDL-C are raised, it undergoes a process called oxidation and is then taken up into the wall of the artery, where it forms plaque. This may lead to arterial narrowing and symptoms of heart disease. For this reason LDL-C is often referred to as the 'bad cholesterol'.

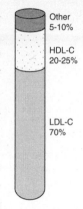

Figure 20

HDL-C, on the other hand, normally carries about 20-25 per cent of the cholesterol in the blood and helps to remove the harmful LDL-C from the circulation. Hence it is some-times called 'good cholesterol'. Other lipoproteins carry the remaining five to ten per cent of cholesterol.

*The aim is to have a low level of LDL-C and a high level of HDL-C.*

It is important to understand that the total cholesterol (TC) level is what most doctors refer to when they talk about high or low cholesterol levels. TC is simply the sum of LDL-C, HDL-C and the small amount of cholesterol carried in other lipoproteins. A high TC level increases the risk of a heart attack, simply because it usually reflects high levels of the harmful LDL-C.

## How is cholesterol measured?

Cholesterol levels – TC, LDL-C and HDL-C – and triglycerides (see p.108) are measured by a blood test. This may involve taking blood with a needle and syringe and sending the sample to a laboratory, or a finger prick (capillary) sample can be taken and analysed on a special desktop analyser. The results of the tests are expressed in units called millimoles per litre, normally written as mmol/L.

Average values of TC, LDL-C, HDL-C and triglycerides for women in the UK, together with the recommended levels, are shown below. *You can see that the optimal or recommended level for TC is less than 5 mmol/L.*

*Table 6*  Cholesterol levels for women in the UK

| Measurement | Average UK values (mmol/L) | Recommended levels (mmol/L) |
| --- | --- | --- |
| Total Cholesterol | 5.8 | Less than 5 |
| LDL-cholesterol | 3.8 | Less than 3 |
| HDL-cholesterol | 1.6 | Above 1 |
| Triglycerides | 1.1 | Less than 2 |

*Recommended levels are based on the latest European Guidelines (1998)

## Which measure is the best indicator of risk?

As we saw earlier, increased levels of LDL-C are associated with an increased risk of heart disease, whereas high levels of HDL-C are strongly protective. Given that the TC level is (mainly) the sum of LDL-C and HDL-C, it is not always a good indicator of heart attack risk when used alone. Clearly, what matters is not simply your total cholesterol level, but rather *how much* is carried in the form of LDL-C and how much as HDL-C. If your TC is mainly in the form of LDL-C, then clearly your risk will be high. Conversely, if your TC has a large proportion of HDL-C, your risk will be low.

To take this into account, doctors often use the ratio between TC and HDL-C – that is, they divide the total cholesterol level by the HDL-C level (TC/HDL-C). So, for example, if your TC is 6 and your HDL-C is 3, then the TC/HDL-C ratio is 6/3 = 2.

*The TC/HDL-C ratio is the most powerful lipid predictor of all. A ratio of greater than five indicates an increased risk of heart attack and a ratio of less than three indicates a low risk.* To illustrate this point further, Figure 21 (below) shows risks for three non-smoking, non-diabetic women, with the same blood pressure (130/80 mmHg) and with TC levels of 6.0 mmol/L. The risk is quite different in each case, simply because, although the TC level is the same for all three, the proportion of LDL-C and HDL-C differs significantly.

*Figure 21*

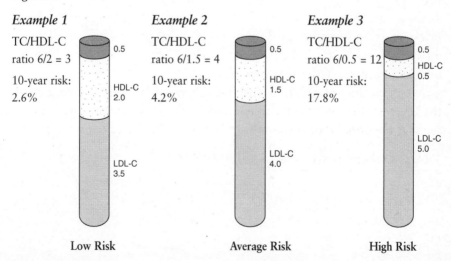

| Example 1 | Example 2 | Example 3 |
|---|---|---|
| TC/HDL-C ratio 6/2 = 3 | TC/HDL-C ratio 6/1.5 = 4 | TC/HDL-C ratio 6/0.5 = 12 |
| 10-year risk: 2.6% | 10-year risk: 4.2% | 10-year risk: 17.8% |
| Low Risk | Average Risk | High Risk |

**Note:** The small amount of cholesterol carried by other lipoproteins is constant at 0.5 mmol/L

You can now see why a single measurement of cholesterol may have limited use. It also explains why, even if your cholesterol is in the optimal range (less than five), you could still be at increased risk of a heart attack. For example, if your TC is 4.8 but your HDL-C is only 0.5, your TC/HDL-C ratio is 9.6.

Conversely, even if your TC is very high, say 9 mmol/L, if your HDL-C is a healthy 2, the TC/HDL-C ratio is just 4.5 – about average.

### Triglycerides

Another blood lipid to consider is the triglyceride level. Triglycerides are fats that come from your diet or are manufactured by the body. Calories taken in during a meal, which are not used immediately by tissues for energy, are converted to fat cells for storage. In fact, body fat is made up mostly of stored triglycerides and, when the body needs extra energy, these fat stores are used. Although not a significant risk factor in men, raised triglyceride levels in women do appear to increase the risk of coronary heart disease, although not to the same extent as high cholesterol levels. Fasting triglyceride levels greater than 2.0 mmol/L indicate increased risk.

Triglyceride levels are increased by obesity, diabetes, heavy alcohol consumption and high sugar intake.

## What factors influence blood cholesterol levels?

**Age and sex:** As we saw in Chapter 3, cholesterol levels (TC & LDL-C) increase with age in both sexes. Until the age of 55, levels tend to be higher in men, but thereafter they tend to be higher in women, except in those taking hormone replacement therapy. In addition, the number of women with cholesterol levels greater than 7 mmol/L rises dramatically in middle-age (see Figure 22).

*Figure 22*   Total cholesterol >7 mmol/L by age group

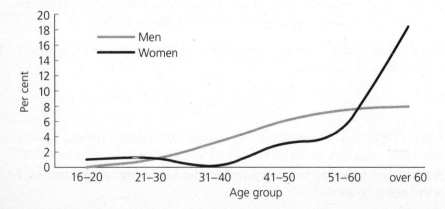

**Dietary fat:** The most common cause of high blood cholesterol levels in people in the UK is too much fat in the diet. TC and LDL-C levels tend to rise and HDL-C levels tend to fall with the amount of saturated fats eaten. Consequently, populations which consume diets rich in saturated fats have high rates of coronary heart disease. Foods rich in saturated fat include butter, fatty meats, full-fat dairy products, fast foods and pastries. The more of these foods you eat, the higher your cholesterol levels are likely to be. Reducing your intake of saturated fats is central to any cholesterol-lowering strategy.

**Being overweight:** Being overweight tends to be associated with high blood cholesterol and triglyceride levels, usually because of excessive intake of dietary fats. Being overweight also tends to lower levels of HDL-C, further increasing the risk of heart disease.

**Physical activity:** Many people are under the impression that exercise lowers cholesterol levels, but this is not the case. It has little impact on either TC or LDL-C, but it may increase HDL-C levels slightly. Because of the discussion earlier, you can now appreciate that if the LDL-C level does not change as a result of exercise, but the HDL-C levels rises, there may be an *increase* in TC.

**Heavy alcohol intake:** People who drink large quantities of alcohol often have abnormal blood lipids, particularly high triglyceride levels.

**Genetic factors:** In the vast majority of cases, high cholesterol levels are due to an excessive intake of saturated fats. However, a small number of people – one in 500 – have an inherited disorder called *familial hyperlipidaemia* or FH. These individuals have very high levels of TC, usually between 9 and 12 mmol/L or even higher. FH is discussed in more detail later in this section.

**Other diseases:** Other physical conditions can result in high cholesterol levels, including thyroid and kidney disease and diabetes.

**Drugs:** Some prescribed drugs, e.g. diuretics, beta blockers and oral contraceptives, may have unfavourable effects on blood lipids.

Most of these factors, though not all, are readily modifiable by relatively modest lifestyle changes.

# Action plan

High cholesterol levels don't usually cause any symptoms, unless you have already developed heart problems as a result. As with blood pressure, the only way to know whether you have a high cholesterol level is to have it measured.

## Where should I have my lipids measured?

The easiest option is to arrange for the test with your family doctor, although some GPs are more receptive than others. Nowadays, doctors are being encouraged to be become more proactive where prevention is concerned and many surgeries have practice nurses who can do the test for you. Moreover, if you have already had a heart attack or symptoms of angina, your blood lipids will have been measured as a matter of course. An overnight fast before having the blood test is recommended, because eating tends to increase triglyceride levels. However, contrary to what you may have been told, you do not need to be in the fasting state if only cholesterol measurements are being made.

If you don't want to ask your own doctor to measure your lipids, many private healthcare organisations will arrange the tests for you, although this is usually only a small component of a much more comprehensive (and expensive) assessment. Some retail pharmacy outlets also offer cholesterol and blood pressure testing, usually using what are referred to as 'dry chemistry analysers'. A finger prick sample is all that is required and the results should be available in just a few minutes. Provided that the instruments are carefully calibrated and the operator has been well trained, the results are reliable. However, they may only offer TC measurement, rather than TC and HDL-C. You may also have seen cholesterol 'self-test' kits in some chemist shops. These involve puncturing the end of your own finger, spreading a small amount of blood onto the test paper and reading the result from a colour chart after a minute or two. These tests are unreliable and best avoided.

## A cholesterol-lowering diet

People are sometimes confused about the difference between a cholesterol-lowering diet and a low-cholesterol diet, and the difference *is* important. Let me explain.

Although it will probably seem strange, it is the amount of saturated fat, not cholesterol, in the diet, which has the largest effect on your blood cholesterol level. Cholesterol-rich foods such as kidneys, liver and eggs actually have a relatively small effect on blood cholesterol levels, because they contain only small amounts of saturated fat. An article in the prestigious *New England Journal of Medicine* entitled 'Normal Plasma Cholesterol In An 88-Year-Old-Man Who Eats 25 Eggs a Day' illustrates my point! This is not to say that dietary cholesterol can be ignored if you are trying to lower your blood cholesterol, only that the saturated fat content is more important (NB. for a fuller discussion of fats, including trans fats, see p.112).

In theory, therefore, you could follow a low cholesterol diet, but if the saturated fat content were high, your blood cholesterol level wouldn't improve very much. Conversely, consuming cholesterol-rich foods which are nonetheless low in saturated fat, may still lower your blood cholesterol. So, the key to getting your cholesterol down is to pursue a cholesterol-lowering diet, i.e. one low in saturated fats, rather than a low-cholesterol diet which may or may not be low in saturated fat.

The principles of reducing your daily saturated fat intake are simple:

---

### A CHOLESTEROL-LOWERING DIET

✓ Eat fish, poultry without the skin, and leaner cuts of meat (trim the visible fat away)

✓ Eat fewer high-fat processed meats, such as sausage, meat pies, salami, luncheon meat and hot dogs

✓ Limit your consumption of cheese, cream, eggs and other dairy products which tend to be high in saturated fat

✓ Drink less whole milk and substitute either semi-skimmed or skimmed milk (which are actually richer sources of calcium)

✓ Increase your consumption of fresh vegetables and fruit and try to eat a purely vegetarian meal once or twice a week

✓ Avoid creamy dressings or sauces – look for low-fat or oil free dressings

✓ Eat more cereals, bread, pasta and other wholegrain products

✓ Reduce your intake of chocolates, cakes, pastries and biscuits which tend to contain large amounts of saturated fat and *trans* fats

✓ Try to use the frying pan less often; grill, bake or boil instead. Microwave cooking is particularly helpful. If you do fry, then use a monounsaturated oil (e.g. olive oil, rapeseed oil) or a polyunsaturated oil (e.g. safflower oil, sunflower oil)

✓ Include foods which are high in soluble fibre – oats, peas, beans, lentils and apples – as these may have a modest cholesterol-lowering effect

✓ Consider using Benecol spreads and (possibly) Olestra products

---

See Appendix 2, p.234, for more specific information on food choices for lowering cholesterol.

## What about trans fats? . . .

Many people believe that by substituting polyunsaturated margarines for butter, they will help to reduce their cholesterol levels. However, some hard margarines can actually increase the 'bad' LDL-C and lower the 'good' HDL-C. This is because they contain *trans* fats, which are a by-product of an industrial process called hydrogenation. Hydrogenation involves taking unsaturated fats and adding hydrogen to them, so that they become firmer at room temperature and less likely to go rancid. The more solid the margarine, the more trans fatty acids it contains, whereas softer margarines contain smaller amounts of trans fats. Since trans fats can increase LDL-C and lower HDL-C, it is no surprise to find that they increase the risk of coronary heart disease.

Trans fats are found naturally, albeit in small quantities, in some dairy foods and meat, but the majority come from margarines (especially hard margarines), fried foods, cakes, pastries, biscuits and savoury snacks. Because food labels contain no information about the content of trans fats, it is best to limit your intake by avoiding these foods and by choosing margarine labelled as 'trans free'.

## . . . and Olestra and Benecol?

Two products which have received a lot of media coverage, Olestra and Benecol could also contribute to a cholesterol-lowering diet. But do they?

**Olestra,** a fat substitute, was developed to meet increasing consumer demand for low-fat snack foods that taste like the real thing. It is actually made from sucrose and fat, but they are combined in such a way that the body cannot break them apart. Therefore, Olestra is not absorbed by the body and contributes no calories.

Olestra can be used to imitate the 'mouth feel' of familiar snack foods – so you can get the taste without the guilt! For example, a 30 gram (1oz) bag of crisps made with Olestra contains 0g of fat and about 70 calories, compared with 10g of fat and 150 calories for the same quantity of full-fat crisps. Olestra has been under development for around 30 years, has undergone extensive testing and appears to be safe. There is, incidentally, no evidence to suggest any significant interaction between Olestra products and commonly prescribed medications.

Sounds great, but there have been two major concerns about Olestra. The first is that Olestra might reduce the absorption into the body of important fat-soluble vitamins – vitamins A,D,E,K and some carotenoids. However, the effect is small and research shows that it can be offset by adding each of the four fat-soluble vitamins to Olestra products, which is precisely what the manufacturers now do. The effect on carotenoids is also very small and supplements are not required. Olestra cannot affect any vitamins or carotenoids already stored in the body.

The more familiar, less theoretical problem is Olestra's effects on the digestive system – including stomach cramps, loose motions, bloating and nausea. However, recent research shows that these symptoms are actually no more common in those consuming Olestra products than in those eating the usual, full-fat versions.

So what help will Olestra be to you? Firstly, if you are trying to lose weight as part of your cholesterol-lowering programme, Olestra can help to reduce your daily calorie intake. Please be aware, however, that because Olestra products are fat-free, they are not calorie-free. This is because the fat in the product is replaced by carbohydrate or protein, both of which contain four calories per gram (rather than the nine calories per gram from fat). Evidence shows that Olestra products can help individuals to lose weight, by providing a wider choice of lower-fat snacks. Secondly, as far as cholesterol-lowering is concerned, the contribution of Olestra is likely to be very small and, in most cases, insignificant.

**Benecol** margarine contains a unique cholesterol-lowering ingredient known as plant stanol ester, which works by inhibiting cholesterol absorption through the intestine. Studies show that Benecol can lower TC and LDL-cholesterol by up to 14 per cent, without any detrimental effect on HDL-C or triglycerides. Benecol spreads come in regular and light versions, though both contain the same amount of plant stanol ester. The regular Benecol spread can be used in cooking like any other margarine or on bread, but the light spread is meant to be used only on bread. Additional Benecol products include cream cheese style spreads and fruit yogurts.

Since Benecol products appear to be quite safe, they can be built into an overall diet for cholesterol-lowering, although they are not usually recommended for children or pregnant women. They can also be used quite safely with cholesterol-lowering medication.

## What about eating out?

Sticking to a cholesterol-lowering diet if you eat out a lot will not be easy. It is, therefore, very important to make sure that your diet at home is right and then, when you do eat out, choose something from the menu that represents the best compromise in terms of its fat content. Tips for eating out are given in Appendix 3, p.236.

## What about familial hyperlipidaemia (FH)?

In this inherited condition, which is found in about one in 500 people in Britain, the mechanism by which LDL-C is removed from the blood circulation works only half as effectively as normal. This means that people with FH have cholesterol levels approximately twice the normal, i.e. 9–12 mmol/L.

FH is a 'dominantly inherited' disorder, which means that if you have FH, your brothers, sisters and your own children will each have a 50/50 chance of having FH too.

If you have the condition, your doctor will usually arrange to check other members of the family. If someone in your immediate family has FH, or a history of heart disease in their 50s, you should have your lipids measured. Don't be put off from asking to have this done just because you feel perfectly well; many people with FH are not obese and may not have any other obvious risk factors.

The main problem with FH is that the condition leads to heart problems at a relatively early age, usually before 60. Although FH affects men and women equally, its impact on heart disease is rather different. Without treatment, over half the men with FH will die before their sixtieth birthday. Untreated women do rather better, with about one in seven dying before they reach 60. Even at the age of 70, some untreated women are still free from heart trouble, whereas this would be unusual in a man. So a man who inherits FH from his mother may actually develop heart disease long before she does.

The treatment of FH is really no different from that of the more usual causes of high cholesterol. Although it is very important to stick to a cholesterol-lowering diet, diet alone is unlikely to be enough and you will need to take cholesterol-lowering drugs too. Children with FH may also need medication if there is a strong family history of heart disease. For these reasons, your doctor will probably refer you to a specialist to ensure that you get the most appropriate treatment.

You can get more information on FH from your doctor or the Family Heart Association (see Appendix 1, p.227).

## Will I need cholesterol-lowering drugs?

This depends upon your overall risk of coronary disease as well as your TC and LDL-C level. The higher your risk of heart disease, the more likely it is that your doctor will want to prescribe lipid-lowering drugs. Those at highest risk are:

- Those who have already had a heart attack.
- Those who have angina.
- Those who have had bypass surgery or angioplasty.

Your doctor will normally ask you to follow a low-fat diet for a period of three to six months before considering the addition of drugs. Remember, even if your doctor prescribes cholesterol-lowering drugs, you must still follow a cholesterol-lowering diet and pay close attention to other risk factors such as stopping smoking, taking regular exercise and controlling your weight. More detailed information about cholesterol-lowering drugs can be found in Chapter 5.

## What should my cholesterol goal be?

Based on the latest guidelines, you should aim for a total cholesterol of less than 5.0 mmol/L and an LDL-C of less than 3.0 mmol/L.

## How long will it take to lower my cholesterol?

There is a great deal of individual variation in terms of a response to a cholesterol-lowering diet. Generally, both total cholesterol and LDL-C should begin to fall two to three weeks after you begin your cholesterol-lowering diet. How much you reduce your blood cholesterol levels depends on how much fat you were eating before starting the cholesterol-lowering diet, how well you stick to the diet and how responsive your body is to the change in fat intake. Also, the higher your blood cholesterol is to begin with, the greater the reduction you can expect. Over time, you may reduce your cholesterol by 1 to 1.5 mmol/L or even more. Your doctor will want to measure your lipids after you have been on the diet for four to six weeks and then again after three to six months. If you have achieved your cholesterol goal, you will probably have your lipids measured twice a year thereafter.

If your doctor starts you on cholesterol-lowering drugs in addition to dietary measures, you can expect an even greater reduction in cholesterol levels over a shorter time. Normally your doctor will measure your lipids about four weeks after starting treatment, and then at regular intervals until an adequate response to drug therapy has been confirmed.

## How long will treatment last?

Your cholesterol-lowering diet, with or without drug therapy, should be continued for life. The occasional piece of chocolate cake or sticky toffee pudding won't do any harm, but resuming your old eating habits may. The problem is that making excuses for 'special occasions' can become just a bit too easy. In fact, you will be surprised at how quickly your new eating patterns will become part of your normal routine, without seeming to be a special diet at all.

## What about triglycerides?

We saw earlier in this section that elevated triglycerides are an important risk factor for heart disease in women. High triglyceride levels are usually seen in combination with high levels of total cholesterol and LDL-cholesterol and so respond to the same dietary and lifestyle changes referred to earlier in this section, i.e. a diet low in saturated fat, weight loss (if overweight), and increased physical activity. In those who are not obese, saturated fat should be replaced by monounsaturated and polyunsaturated fats.

Studies have shown that large doses of fish-oil supplements, which are rich in omega-3 fatty acids, can lower triglycerides by 1 mmol/L. Although supplements may be appropriate for those with very high triglyceride levels, for most people a regular consumption of fish rich in omega-3s – mackerel, sardines canned in oil, herring, salmon, lake trout, tuna and anchovies – combined with other dietary measures, is enough.

High triglyceride levels are also associated with heavy alcohol intake and diabetes, so ensuring that your alcohol consumption is within safe-drinking guidelines and that your diabetes is well controlled is also important. Certain drugs, for example fibrates, are particularly effective at reducing triglyceride levels and may be appropriate for some individuals.

## Will lowering my cholesterol reduce my risk of heart disease?

Yes, most definitely. Studies show that for each one per cent reduction in cholesterol, there is a two to three per cent reduction in risk and this is particularly true for those who already have a history of coronary heart disease. Under normal circumstances you can expect that dietary measures alone will reduce your cholesterol and LDL-C by about 10 per cent, which means that you can reduce your risk of heart problems by about 20–30 per cent. Drugs may produce an even larger reduction in cholesterol, and so may reduce the risk of heart disease by an even larger amount.

The key points from this Action File are summarized below.

## KEY POINTS TO LOWER YOUR CHOLESTEROL

- Follow a diet low in saturated fat and *trans* fats but high in fresh fruit and vegetables, fish, cereals, pasta and wholegrain foods
- Consider using Olestra and Benecol products
- Maintain a healthy weight and take regular, moderate exercise
- Keep your alcohol intake within sensible limits
- Take cholesterol-lowering drugs as prescribed
- Have your cholesterol and other lipids checked regularly

# Controlling your blood pressure

This Action File is all about getting – and keeping – your blood pressure under control. High blood pressure, or hypertension, is a common and extremely important condition which affects about a third of women aged 16 years and over. Hypertension greatly increases the risk of stroke and coronary heart disease in women, particularly in those aged 60 and over. It may cause enlargement of the heart (left ventricular hypertrophy), leading to heart failure. Apart from the heart and brain, hypertension can also damage the arteries supplying the eyes and the kidneys, leading to deteriorating vision and kidney failure. Put simply, the higher your blood pressure, the shorter your life expectancy. Fortunately, there is an enormous amount that you can do to lower your blood pressure. It takes only modest changes in lifestyle, sometimes combined with modern drug therapy, to get your blood pressure down – and keep it there!

## Background

As we saw in Chapter 3, blood pressure simply refers to the pressure of blood in the arteries. A certain amount of blood pressure is needed to keep the blood flowing through the arteries and is, therefore, essential to life. This may seem a very elementary point, but the fact is that many people are confused by the term 'blood pressure' and are under the impression that blood pressure at any level is harmful. This is not the case. Blood pressure is only harmful if it becomes too high, usually as a consequence of the arteries losing their normal elasticity.

### How is blood pressure measured?

The instrument used to measure blood pressure is called a sphygmomanometer (you will almost certainly have seen this sitting on your doctor's desk). It consists of an inflatable cuff which is placed around your arm and a tube of mercury which measures the pressure. Blood pressure is measured in millimetres of mercury (mm Hg), with one number over the other, e.g. 120/80 mmHg. The higher of the two readings (120) is the systolic blood pressure (SBP), which is the pressure in the arteries when the heart is contracting. The lower of the two readings (80) is the diastolic blood pressure (DBP), which is the pressure when the heart is resting between beats.

Your own doctor or the practice nurse will be happy to measure your blood pressure for you. It takes only a few moments and is completely painless. Some retail chemist shops also offer a blood pressure testing service.

## How do we define normal and high blood pressure?

In Chapter 3, high blood pressure was defined as a systolic blood pressure (SBP) of 140 mmHg or greater and/or a diastolic blood pressure (DBP) of 90 mmHg or greater. Put another way, we can say that normal blood pressure (BP) for adults is 139/89 mmHg or below.

However, there is no fixed dividing line between normal pressure and slightly raised blood pressure. Table 7 shows the classification of different levels of BP according to the most recent guidelines.

*Table 7*  Blood pressure classification (mmHg)

| Category | Systolic | Diastolic |
| --- | --- | --- |
| *Normal* | | |
| Optimal (Ideal) | < 120 | < 80 |
| Normal | < 130 | < 85 |
| High Normal | 130–139 | 85–89 |
| *Hypertension* | | |
| Grade 1 (mild) | 140–159 | 90–99 |
| Grade 2 (moderate) | 160–179 | 100–109 |
| Grade 3 (severe) | ≥180 | ≥110 |

NB.   < means less than
        ≥ means greater than or equal to

## Does blood pressure vary?

Blood pressure varies considerably throughout the day and night. During sleep, when all our various bodily systems are relatively inactive and the demand for oxygen is low, blood pressure falls. The lowest readings tend to be in the early hours of the morning and then, between 6 and 8a.m., the pressure begins to rise again. Stress, driving a car in heavy traffic, eating, alcohol and physical activity, can all affect blood pressure levels during a 24-hour period.

Given that blood pressure in the normal state can vary so widely, how is it possible to make a reliable diagnosis of high blood pressure? The answer is that doctors always try to standardise their measurements by taking the blood pressure in a resting state, usually with the patient reclining on a couch. Even then, the readings may vary quite a bit from one visit to the next. This is why your doctor will ask you back two or three times before deciding whether your blood pressure is normal or high.

Some people seem to have an aversion to having their blood pressure measured; the moment the doctor places the cuff around the arm, their heart rate and blood pressure increase dramatically. This is called 'white coat hypertension' (because of its association with the doctor). In recent years modern computer technology has made it possible to measure, record and store blood pressure readings at regular intervals throughout the day, known as 24-hour ambulatory monitoring. Your doctor may use this test if there is any doubt about the diagnosis of hypertension, or to monitor the effects of drug treatment (See Chapter 5).

## What other tests will be done?

If your blood pressure is high, your doctor will usually examine your heart and lungs and generally check for evidence of circulatory problems. This will include feeling pulses in your legs and looking at the backs of your eyes to see if the small blood vessels of the retina show any damage. You will probably have an electrocardiogram (ECG) and a chest X-ray to check if your heart is enlarged. You may also have some simple blood and urine tests to make sure your kidneys are functioning normally.

## What are the symptoms of hypertension?

Many people believe that hypertension causes headaches and other symptoms, but this is not so. Most people who have high blood pressure do not have headaches and most of us with headaches have normal blood pressures. In fact, hypertension only rarely makes people feel ill and in many cases the first evidence of it may be a heart attack or stroke. Because of this it is often referred to as the 'silent killer'. In practice, therefore, the only way to know if your blood pressure is high, is to have it measured.

## How does hypertension lead to heart disease?

The effects of high blood pressure can be divided into two main groups:

- Those due to pressure changes within the heart and arteries.
- Those due to direct arterial damage.

The constant high pressure in the arterial system throws an enormous extra burden on the heart, which is able to compensate in the early stages by developing a thicker muscle wall (a condition known as left ventricular hypertrophy). Eventually, however, even a thickened heart muscle is not able to overcome the increased pressure in the arterial system, and it begins to fail. The patient begins to notice increasing breathlessness, initially on exertion, but later, also at rest. If this continues untreated, the symptoms of heart failure will become more severe as the heart muscle becomes progressively weaker.

Direct damage to the arteries leads to an acceleration of plaque formation, particularly in those who smoke or have high blood cholesterol. Exactly how or why this occurs is not clear.

## What causes hypertension?

In most cases of high blood pressure, the cause cannot be identified and we refer to this form of high blood pressure as 'primary' or 'essential' hypertension. In practice this accounts for the vast majority – about 90 per cent – of patients with hypertension. Of course, certain lifestyle-related factors such as being overweight, physical inactivity, heavy alcohol and salt consumption, make a major contribution to this form of hypertension. It is also true to say that hypertension tends to run in families, so that if your mother and father were hypertensive, you are more likely to develop high blood pressure yourself. Part of this may be due to the fact that children tend to inherit the bad health habits of their parents, such as poor diet and obesity. But there also appears to be an independent genetic factor involved, which may make some individuals more sensitive to salt and, therefore, more prone to hypertension (see p.124).

In the remaining 10 per cent, there is an underlying cause which can be identified and these cases are referred to as secondary, i.e. the high blood pressure is secondary to some underlying disease – most often of the kidneys – although in rare cases it may also be due to certain tumours or drugs. However, the two most common causes of secondary hypertension in women are oral contraception and pregnancy.

### Oral contraception
Oral contraceptives contain a combination of oestrogen and progestogen and may interfere with the kidney mechanisms involved in blood pressure regulation, producing a slight rise in blood pressure. However, some women may be particularly sensitive to the Pill and develop hypertension.

This is why, if you are taking oral contraception, your doctor will wish to check your blood pressure at regular intervals. Because the rise in blood pressure tends to be greater on the higher-dose pill preparations, you should check that you are on a low-dose pill (low-dose pills should be prescribed unless there is a special reason not to). If you do become hypertensive on the Pill, you should stop taking it and use an alternative method of contraception (or a lower dose preparation). You can expect your blood pressure to return to normal within two to three months. (Incidentally, hormone replacement therapy [HRT] is not usually associated with any significant change in blood pressure.)

### Pregnancy

A rise in blood pressure after the twentieth week of pregnancy is one of the signs of a complication known as *pre-eclamptic toxaemia*, or pre-eclampsia. If this happens you may be admitted to hospital for bed rest.

A small elevation of blood pressure towards the end of pregnancy is more common and is usually temporary. However, there is some evidence that women whose blood pressure rises in this way may be more prone to developing hypertension in later life.

## What is Isolated Systolic Hypertension (ISH)?

Isolated systolic hypertension is a form of high blood pressure in older people in which the top number of the reading (SBP) is greater than 160 mmHg while the bottom number (DBP) is in the normal range – that is, below 90 mmHg. In the past, doctors and patients tended to think that ISH was a milder form of blood pressure and, therefore, less dangerous than when both SBP *and* DBP were elevated. However, recent evidence shows that ISH – as with the more usual form of hypertension – is associated with an increased risk of stroke, heart attack and heart failure. Hence, early identification and treatment – usually beginning with a diuretic (water tablet) – is now strongly advised.

## What about hypotension (low blood pressure)?

Having hypotension or low blood pressure (below 110/60) is generally a good thing, since you are likely to live longer than people with high or even 'normal' blood pressure levels. As with high blood pressure, people with hypotension have few symptoms and are usually unaware of it. Occasionally, however, low blood pressure can cause symptoms such as dizziness or fainting, particularly if you stand up quickly after sitting or lying down – known as *postural hypotension*. This tends to be more common in older people in whom the normal bodily mechanisms for keeping blood pressure within certain limits become sluggish. Getting up slowly – so that the body has time to adjust to the new position, usually does the trick and only a very small number of patients will need medication. Hypotension may sometimes be a side-effect of medication used to treat high blood pressure.

# Action plan

If your blood pressure is high, there is a great deal you can do to reduce it to a more acceptable level. In fact, perhaps as many as 80 per cent of individuals with borderline or mild hypertension can reduce their blood pressure to safer levels without resorting to the use of drugs. So what are the practical things that you can do to get your blood pressure down?

**Watch your weight – dropping pounds drops pressure:** There is a strong association between being overweight and having high blood pressure. Fat cells stimulate the production of insulin which helps the body absorb sugar and, therefore, calories. Insulin has other effects, however, and may raise blood pressure by causing the body to retain salt and water. Whatever the mechanism, there is good evidence that shedding the pounds will help lower your blood pressure. For example, a 10 per cent weight loss may reduce both SBP and DBP by as much as 10 mmHg, which may mean the difference between needing and not needing drugs to control blood pressure. Losing weight is discussed in Action File 5, p.150.

**Limit your alcohol intake:** Moderate drinking has a protective effect on the heart in women aged 50 and over, and in men aged 40 and above. However, heavy drinking tends to increase blood pressure levels, leading to a higher risk of heart disease and stroke. By keeping your consumption within the safe drinking guidelines (up to 14 units/week) you can achieve the benefits of moderate drinking without incurring the excess risks of over-consumption. For every unit of alcohol you drink above this upper limit, your SBP is likely to increase by 1 mmHg.

**Exercise regularly:** There is ample scientific evidence to suggest that women who are physically active have lower blood pressure levels than those who are sedentary. If you are hypertensive, moderately intense exercise training can lower your systolic blood pressure by as much as 10–15 mmHg and your diastolic by 8–10 mmHg, an effect which can be achieved without the need for dietary alterations or even weight reduction. However, if your blood pressure is low or normal prior to training, regular exercise will probably have little effect on it.

The type of exercise is important. Aerobic exercises such as swimming, jogging, brisk walking and cycling are fine, but exercises such as weight training which have a large isometric component do not lower blood pressure. On the contrary, they may increase blood pressure to quite dangerous levels. If you have high blood pressure, therefore, avoid weight training and other strength exercises.

For the vast majority of people with hypertension, exercise is both safe and beneficial. Recommended forms of exercise are those which are regular, rhythmical and involve large muscle groups, such as brisk walking, cycling and swimming. If possible, aim for 30 minutes on most days of the week. If you are currently sedentary, a good starting point is a graded walking programme. If you are overweight, then a non-weight-bearing exercise such as swimming or the use of a stationary exercise bicycle for four or five 30-minute sessions per week, has much to recommend it. Remember, too, that some drugs used for the treatment of hypertension will limit your heart rate during exercise and this will need to be taken into account if you are using your pulse rate to monitor your exercise session. Exercise is discussed in more detail in Action File 4, p.131.

Finally, do not ignore symptoms such as chest pain, dizziness or undue breathlessness associated with your exercise session: stop exercising immediately and seek medical advice.

**Reduce your salt consumption:** There is a strong link between high salt intake and high blood pressure, although precisely why this should be the case is still not entirely clear. Every molecule of common table salt (sodium chloride) is made up of one atom of sodium and one atom of chloride, but it is the sodium which contributes to high blood pressure. It seems that people with hypertension have an inability to handle heavy sodium loads, a characteristic which may well be genetically inherited and which may go some way to explaining why high blood pressure has a tendency to run in families.

Most of us consume many times more salt than we need. An adult needs only about 1g of salt per day, but the average British diet contains about 10 times this amount. Much of this salt is 'hidden' in heavily processed foods such as tinned meats, bottled sauces, crisps, bacon, salad dressings, pizzas and hamburgers. It has been estimated that reducing the amount of salt added to processed foods would lower blood pressure levels sufficiently to prevent some 70,000 deaths a year in Britain, as well as much disability. Of course, the difficulty lies in persuading food manufacturers to lower the large amounts of salt added to foods during the production process.

If you have high blood pressure, you would be well advised to cut down on your salt consumption. You should be able to achieve this quite easily by:

- Cutting out salt in cooking and at the table.
- Using more fresh (unprocessed) produce.
- Avoiding highly salted foods such as cooked meats (salami, ham, etc.), salted nuts, crisps, pickles, some cheeses, smoked fish, anchovies, hamburgers, stock cubes and certain sauces such as ketchup and soy sauce.
- Using a salt substitute (usually a potassium salt) available from most chemist shops.
- Using a wider variety of herbs and spices as a substitute for salt in your cooking.
- Reading food labels and choosing low-sodium products. The amount of sodium is shown as the number of grams (g) per 100g of product. The guidelines are:
  - Sodium (salt) free: contains less than 0.005g (5mg) per 100g
  - Very low sodium: contains less than 0.035g (35mg) per 100g
  - Low sodium: contains less than 0.14g (140mg) per 100g

(Just for comparison, a well known form of pickle contains 1.6g [1600mg] of sodium per 100g – not too good if you're trying to cut down on salt!)

You may think that you can't possibly get used to salt-free food, but you will surprise yourself. Within a couple of months your taste will have adjusted and you may actually begin to dislike salty foods.

**Reducing stress:** Emotional upset and other forms of mental stress can increase blood pressure levels, at least in the short term. The mere process of walking into your doctor's surgery can be sufficient to provoke a rapid rise in blood pressure. Whether more prolonged stress and anxiety can contribute to a permanent increase in blood pressure levels is unclear. In the Framingham Heart Study (see p.28), anxiety was a strong predictor of hypertension in middle-aged men, but not in women. But even if stress does not contribute to hypertension, there is evidence that relaxation techniques, including yoga, biofeedback and transcendental meditation, can produce a moderate, but sustained, fall in blood pressure. Reductions of at least 5–10 mmHg are quite possible, without adverse side-effects –

a very worthwhile strategy. Stress management is discussed in more detail in Action File 7, p.187.

**Eat foods containing potassium, calcium and magnesium and fish oils:** In recent years a great deal of research has been carried out into the effects of various dietary factors in controlling blood pressure. There is some evidence that increasing your consumption of potassium-rich foods, such as orange and tomato juice, bananas and other fresh fruits can help. Foods rich in calcium and magnesium may also be beneficial and are discussed below in the DASH diet.

Fish oils have a variety of potentially beneficial effects on the blood, including a lowering of triglycerides, an increase in HDL-cholesterol and a reduced tendency of the blood to clot, all of which contribute to a lower risk of heart attack. However, there is also some evidence that regular consumption of oily fish may help to reduce blood pressure in some individuals. For these reasons and others, regular consumption of fish is strongly recommended.

## The DASH diet

The DASH (Dietary Approaches to Stop Hypertension) was a US-based research study designed to test the effect of various diets on blood pressure. The results of this study, published in 1997, showed that a diet low in total and saturated fat and rich in fruits, vegetables and low-fat dairy foods, can significantly lower blood pressure. In patients who were already hypertensive, the DASH diet lowered blood pressure to the same extent as anti-hypertensive drugs.

The DASH diet consists of six main food groups:

*Grains and grain products, including breads and cereals.* Important sources of energy, fibre and vitamins. Choose whole grains such as wholemeal bread and whole-grain cereals to obtain most of the nutrients.

*Vegetables*: Vegetables such as potatoes, peas, carrots, broccoli and beans are rich sources of potassium, magnesium and fibre.

*Fruits and juices*: Important sources of potassium, magnesium and fibre and are naturally low in sodium and fat. Fresh, frozen, tinned and dried fruits can all be used.

*Low-fat dairy foods*: Major sources of protein and calcium. It is important to select low-fat products to reduce your total daily fat consumption.

*Meat, poultry and fish*: Good sources of high quality protein and magnesium.

*Nuts, seeds and legumes*: Rich sources of energy, magnesium, potassium, protein and fibre. Nuts and seeds are also high in fat, so portions should be small.

The DASH diet is shown on p.128. Please remember, however, that the number of servings applies to people who need 2000 calories per day. The number of servings may increase or decrease depending on your calorie requirements, which will vary according to age, body weight and physical activity patterns. The key point is that the *proportions* of each food group consumed must be maintained.

Here are some tips on DASH eating:

- Start small and keep it simple. Most people find it hard to make changes in their diet if they do too much too fast, so make the changes gradually. That way you are more likely to maintain your healthier eating habits.
- Treat meat as just one part of the meal, not the main focus. Although meat contains protein and other important nutrients, it also tends to have quite a bit of fat, calories and cholesterol.
- Make carbohydrates such as pasta, rice, beans, and vegetables the main focus of your meal.
- Use fresh fruits or low-fat, low-calorie yogurts for sweets.
- Keep a diary. It's much easier to see what's happening with your diet when you write it down, particularly in the early stages of adapting to new eating patterns.
- Make the DASH diet a part of an overall lifestyle that includes reducing your salt and alcohol intake, becoming more physically active and (if necessary) losing weight.

If you are taking tablets for high blood pressure, you must continue taking these as normal. Don't just stop the medication and start the diet. Discuss the idea with your doctor first (see p.129).

For many people, the lifestyle measures described above may well be enough to lower their blood pressure to an acceptable level. For others, some form of drug treatment may also be required. But do please remember that drug treatment is not instead of, but in addition to lifestyle measures. Making lifestyle changes may well reduce the dosage of drugs required to control your blood pressure, and will have additional cardiovascular benefits.

*Table 8*  The DASH diet

| Food group | No of servings | Serving sizes | Examples and notes | Significance to the DASH diet |
|---|---|---|---|---|
| Grains and grain products | 7–8 per day | 1 slice bread<br>56g (2 oz) dry cereal<br>56g (2 oz) cooked rice, pasta, or cereal | whole-wheat bread, English muffin, pitta bread, bagel, cereals, oatmeal | major sources of energy and fibre |
| Vegetables | 4–5 per day | 112g (4 oz) raw leafy vegetable<br>56g (2 oz) cooked vegetable<br>170ml (6 floz) vegetable juice | tomatoes, potatoes, carrots, peas, squash, broccoli, turnip greens, kale, spinach, artichokes, beans, sweet potatoes | rich sources of potassium, magnesium and fibre |
| Fruits | 4–5 per day | 170ml (6 floz) fruit juice<br>1 medium fruit<br>28g (1 oz) dried fruit<br>56g (2 oz) fresh, frozen, or canned fruit | apricots, bananas, dates, grapes, oranges, orange juice, grapefruit, grapefruit juice, mangoes, melons, peaches, pineapples, prunes, raisins, strawberries, tangerines | important sources of potassium, magnesium and fibre |
| Low-fat or non-fat dairy foods | 2–3 per day | 220ml (8 floz) milk<br>110ml (4 floz) yoghurt<br>42g (1½ oz) cheese | skimmed or 1% milk, skimmed or low-fat buttermilk, non-fat or low-fat yogurt, part-skimmed mozzarella cheese, non-fat cheese | major sources of calcium and protein |
| Meats, poultry, fish | 2 or less per day | 84g (3 oz) cooked meats, poultry, or fish | select only lean; trim away visible fats; grill, roast or boil, instead of frying; remove skin from poultry | rich sources of protein and magnesium |
| Nuts, seeds, legumes | 4–5 per week | 42g (1½ oz) nuts<br>14g (½ oz) or 2 tablespoons seeds<br>56g (2 oz) cooked legumes | almonds, hazelnuts, mixed nuts, peanuts, walnuts, sunflower seeds, kidney beans, lentils | rich sources of energy, magnesium, potassium, protein and fibre |

## Drug treatment for blood pressure – is it for life?

There are many drugs available for the treatment of hypertension and these are reviewed in detail in Chapter 5. If you have been prescribed medication for high blood pressure, it is obviously important to continue with this.

The key question, however, is: Will it be possible for you to stop taking drugs? The answer is a qualified 'Yes'. Sometimes your doctor may decide to give drugs as a temporary protective measure to allow time for lifestyle strategies such as weight loss, salt restriction, exercise and dietary changes to take effect. It may then be possible to reduce the dose of medication or, in some cases, to stop it altogether. But this should only ever be done after consultation with your doctor. The response to lifestyle changes is highly individual and not everyone will respond sufficiently to avoid taking tablets.

## Will controlling my blood pressure lower my risks?

The short answer is 'Yes'. A number of major studies have shown that treating hypertension saves lives by preventing strokes and heart failure. A sustained decrease in your blood pressure of as little as 5–6 mmHg may reduce your risk of having a heart attack by as much as 25 per cent and for stroke by up to 40 per cent.

## What about home blood pressure monitors?

Having the ability to measure your own blood pressure may well be helpful for some, particularly if you have 'white-coat hypertension' (see p.120). For others it tends to make their anxiety even worse – and makes the readings higher. If you decide to invest in a system, you should ask your doctor for advice. Digital electronic monitors are simple to use, but the readings are not always reliable. Make sure you purchase one that is approved and validated for use in the UK.

## Taking control

The 'take-home' message from this section on lowering blood pressure is that what you can do for yourself – in terms of lifestyle choices with respect to diet, exercise and weight loss – really can make a difference. This is especially true if your hypertension is mild, and about 80 per cent of those with high blood pressure are classified as such. Treating millions of people with drugs when relatively simple changes in lifestyle would be at least as effective is an unnecessary waste of valuable resources, not to mention the potential exposure to the side-effects of medication. Even in more severe cases of hypertension, lifestyle changes can make an important contribution by reducing the dose of drugs required to achieve control.

The key points from this Action File are summarized below:

---

### CHECKLIST FOR BLOOD PRESSURE CONTROL

✓ Achieve or maintain a healthy body weight

✓ Keep alcohol intake to below 14 units/week

✓ Take regular, moderate aerobic exercise

✓ Reduce your sodium intake

✓ Learn to relax and control your stress levels

✓ Follow the DASH diet programme

✓ Remember to take your tablets

✓ Have your blood pressure checked regularly

---

# Why exercise?

Physically active women have only half the risk of heart attack compared with sedentary women. In addition to its beneficial effects on the heart and circulation, an active lifestyle reduces the risk of many other chronic diseases, including diabetes, osteoporosis, obesity and some forms of cancer. Those who already have a history of heart problems will also benefit from regular, moderate exercise and reduce their chances of further problems in future. Start with a walking programme and gradually progress to the aerobic activity of your choice. Aim for 30 minutes on most days of the week and follow the guidelines on monitoring the intensity of your exercise. Enjoy your activities – but don't overdo them!

## Background

*If some of the benefits of regular exercise could be procured by any one Medicine, then nothing in the world would be held in more esteem than that Medicine.*

Francis Fuller (1705)

Francis Fuller was clearly a man ahead of his time. In 1705 he published a remarkable book called *Medicina Gymnastica,* a discussion of the medical benefits of physical activity in patients with various diseases, including heart disease. Leafing through the pages of Fuller's book today, one cannot fail to be impressed by his remarkable insight into the relationship between physical activity and health – all the more extraordinary because he was completely unaware of the complex bodily mechanisms by means of which the benefits of exercise are achieved.

Today we understand an enormous amount about the science of exercise and the biochemical and physiological processes involved. We know roughly how much activity is required to achieve health benefits and we know that physical activity is generally quite safe, even for patients with heart disease. So why is it that the majority of us fail to take even the minimum amount of exercise to maintain a healthy heart and circulation?

## Why are we inactive?

Humans have been civilised only within the last 10,000 years or so. For most of our million years on earth, we were nomads and hunters – moving with the game, walking and sometimes running long distances, setting up and breaking camp.

As societies grew and flourished, methods of growing crops and other vegetable food sources were introduced, and agriculture was born. The vast majority of the population were land workers; even as recently as 1900, 60 per cent of the American population lived on farms. Tilling the soil, planting and harvesting the various crops and cutting wood, all involved lifting, pushing, carrying, walking and other forms of exertion. Life was extremely hard and there was little or no time for relaxation.

Today the situation is vastly different. Anyone from a bygone age stepping into the twenty-first century would be struck by the extent to which we have managed to eliminate physical activity from our daily routine. A century ago, a third of the work done in farms and factories was based on muscle power, compared with only about one per cent today. Since the beginning of the twentieth century, we have witnessed the transformation of an essentially rural society into a population of town- and city-dwellers whose lifestyle bears little resemblance to that of their forbears. Modern technology enables us to live with the absolute minimum of physical exercise. The advent of the car is the most obvious example, but there are countless other areas in which technology has left its mark. Lifts and escalators in offices and shops remove the need to negotiate stairs, we sit in our armchairs and flick from one TV station to another, we spend hours sitting in front of a computer screen 'surfing' and we can order our groceries from the 'online' supermarket. In the US there are even golf courses which *require* their members to use an electric cart rather than walk round the course! The paradox is that our soft and feeble bodies are crying out for more activity, while society is engaged in the business of ensuring that we have to do less – with potentially serious health consequences.

## The consequences of inactivity

Physical inactivity is a major risk factor for heart disease. As we saw in Chapter 3, physically active women – even older women – can halve their risk of a heart attack by taking regular, moderate physical exercise, such as 30–45 minutes of brisk walking on three or more occasions per week.

But of course physical inactivity is also related to many other preventable diseases, particularly obesity, diabetes, osteoporosis and lower back pain. Some cancers, particularly of the breast and bowel, also appear to be related to a sedentary lifestyle.

## How unfit are we?

In the early part of the last century, doctors believed in the 'rate of living theory', which basically stated that the heart was genetically programmed to beat a certain number of times and then you were finished. Using them up during exercise was just a quick way to an early grave. Conversely, the less active you were, the longer you could expect to survive. If the results of recent activity surveys are anything to go by, this theory is alive and well! The Allied Dunbar Survey carried out in 1992 revealed the following:

- In terms of physical activity, more than eight out of 10 women fell below their age-appropriate activity level necessary to achieve health benefits.
- Among 16–24 year old women, nine out of 10 were below the target level recommended for achieving health benefits.
- Activity declines markedly with age; among 65–74 year old women, four out of 10 were entirely sedentary. This is another worrying finding, because elderly people respond well to graded exercise programmes, with consequent improvement in muscle strength, mobility and a reduced likelihood of falls, hip fractures and other injuries.
- Sustaining a reasonable walking pace for several minutes on ground level represented severe exertion for older women – more than one in two women aged 55–64 were not fit enough to continue walking on the level at this speed.
- One in two women aged 55–74 years did not have sufficient thigh strength to rise from a chair without using their arms.
- Among women aged 55 and over, one in two did not have sufficient leg strength to climb stairs without using their arms for assistance.

Despite these poor and very worrying findings, more than 80 per cent of women of all ages believed themselves to be fit and the majority (incorrectly) believed that they did enough exercise to keep fit. The huge discrepancy between the perception and the reality may be just mass self-deception, but is more likely to reflect the fact that many people don't actually know what 'healthful' regular exercise is.

Not that we are alone in being in very poor physical shape. Similar surveys in Canada, Australia and the USA give broadly similar results, indicating that the couch potato lifestyle travels well.

## What are the benefits of physical activity?

Now for the good news – the benefits of exercise.

**Lower risk of coronary heart disease:** As we have seen, women who are physically active have about a 50 per cent reduction in risk compared with women who are inactive.

**Stronger heart:** A well-conditioned heart will pump the same amount of blood in 50 beats per minute as the inactive person's heart pumps in 70 to 75 beats. Compared to the well-conditioned heart, the inactive person's heart has to pump up to 15,000 more times per day – more than half a million times each year.

**Lower risk of cancer:** Exercise may help to protect women against various forms of cancer, particularly of the breast, ovary, cervix, uterus and bowel.

**Preservation of bone density:** Osteoporosis is a particular problem in women after the menopause. HRT has been shown to protect women against bone loss, but there is also good evidence that regular, weight-bearing exercise, can help to preserve healthy bone density. Women who remain physically active into old age are much less likely to suffer from osteoporosis.

**Reduced blood pressure:** Physically active women have lower blood pressures than women who are inactive and unfit. This beneficial effect is one of the mechanisms by which exercise helps to protect against heart disease.

**Reduced body weight:** Regular exercise helps to promote fat loss, whilst improving muscular strength and flexibility. By burning calories more efficiently and helping to preserve muscle tissue, regular exercise helps to maintain a healthy body weight.

**Increased HDL-cholesterol:** Exercise has almost no effect on either total cholesterol or LDL-cholesterol, so the idea that you can just 'burn off' excess blood cholesterol isn't true. Exercise does, however, raise the level of HDL-C which – as we have seen – helps to protect against heart disease in women. Although the rise in HDL-C produced by exercise is, on average, quite small, this has a large impact on heart attack risk.

**Reduced clotting tendency:** An increased tendency for blood to coagulate is an important factor in precipitating heart attacks. One measure of the clotting tendency is the level of a substance in the blood called fibrinogen;

the higher the blood fibrinogen, the greater the risk of thrombosis (see Chapter 3). Exercise reduces blood fibrinogen levels, and therefore the risk of heart attack.

Another important factor is the effect of exercise on blood platelets. These are small particles in the blood, which prevent bleeding from cuts or broken blood vessels by clumping together and initiating the formation of a blood clot. Sometimes platelets mistake the fatty plaque inside a diseased coronary artery as a break in the vessel wall which needs plugging, and in doing so precipitate a clot and a heart attack – hence the term coronary thrombosis. Exercise has been shown to reduce platelet stickiness by up to 40 per cent, and thus reduce the risk of a heart attack.

**Reduced risk of diabetes:** Type II diabetes, also known as maturity-onset or non-insulin dependent diabetes (NIDDM – see p.37) usually appears after the age of 40. Unlike those with Type I diabetes, whose bodies do not manufacture any insulin at all, people with NIDDM continue to secrete some insulin, but the body appears to be more resistant to its effects.

Many studies have shown that regular physical activity is associated with a reduced risk of NIDDM. Exercise reduces insulin resistance and helps to restore the body's ability to handle blood sugar normally. Even younger diabetics who use insulin can benefit from regular exercise. Apart from improving their fitness they will tend to see a reduction in their daily insulin requirements. However, exercise can be hazardous if taken too close to an insulin injection and diabetics need to achieve close control over their blood sugar levels if they are to avoid problems.

**Improved aerobic fitness:** Regular exercise – particularly of the aerobic variety – strengthens the heart and improves the efficiency of the heart and lungs. Obviously, if you exercise regularly then your general level of fitness will be much higher than that of a sedentary individual. Not only does this reduce your risk of developing many forms of disease, but it adds immeasurably to the quality of life.

**Reduced stress and improved moods:** Prolonged exposure to stress hormones such as adrenaline, can increase the pulse rate, blood pressure, blood fats and blood sugar and may be harmful to health (See Action File 7, p.187). There is evidence that regular exercise can help to reduce the sudden hormonal surges that are typical of the stress response. In addition, people who take regular exercise report less depression and fatigue and they also have better sleep patterns. Precisely why exercise should have such beneficial psychological effects is not entirely clear, but it seems that a special group of chemicals known as endorphins, play a part in this. These substances have a chemical structure similar to morphine and may, therefore, act as the body's 'natural' pain-killer. Exercise is known to increase endorphin levels and this may explain why exercise improves mood, reduces anxiety and combats the symptoms of pre-menstrual tension.

**Improved sleeping patterns:** Insomnia is an increasingly common complaint (see Action File 7, p.187) and most of us have experienced occasional sleepless nights from time to time. For some people such difficulties can evolve into a chronic sleeping problem. Regular physical exercise can do much to help restore a normal sleeping pattern by promoting more continuous and restful sleep; it should be an integral part of any strategy for dealing with insomnia.

I think you will agree that, by any measure, this is a pretty impressive list of real benefits that you can achieve by regular, moderate exercise.

## What are the risks of exercise?

The benefits of regular exercise in promoting heart health are clear. But what are the risks involved? The two main considerations are heart problems and injuries to the muscles and joints.

### Heart problems
Occasionally someone may develop heart trouble during exercise, or may even die suddenly. Such events are extremely rare, although they frequently attract a disproportionate amount of press interest. In women under 40 years old who die suddenly, the usual cause is an abnormality of the heart – most commonly a structural fault – which has been present from birth. In women over 40, the commonest underlying cause is coronary heart disease. This is why symptoms such as lightheadedness, chest pain and palpitations during exercise, should never be ignored. In general, women who are physically active have a much lower risk of sudden cardiac death than those who are sedentary.

But what about those who already have heart disease? Again, provided that you take things slowly to start with, build up gradually and don't overdo it, exercise is very safe. The greatest risk for the heart patient lies not in exercising – but in *not* exercising!

### Muscles and joints
The most common injuries resulting from exercise are strained ligaments, muscles and joints. These can be avoided by warming up properly before

exercise, and taking time to cool down properly afterwards (p.145). Correct footwear also helps.

**Other problems**

Other potential problems, such as dehydration, heat exhaustion and heat stroke, are very uncommon and usually occur in athletes and others involved in extremely vigorous exercise. Female athletes involved in long distance running may have *amenorrhoea* (complete cessation of menstruation), which may lead to osteoporosis. But overall we can say that the risks of exercise, though not irrelevant, are small and are overwhelmingly outweighed by the benefits.

## What if I already have heart disease?

There was a time when patients who had suffered a heart attack were warned against any kind of exertion, for fear that it would provoke another attack. Today, patients with heart disease are not merely allowed to exercise, they are positively encouraged to do so. Indeed, exercise should form the cornerstone of any cardiac rehabilitation programme. Regular exercise following a heart attack has been shown to improve the function of the heart muscle and to reduce the risks of any further heart problems.

Most patients with heart problems can exercise perfectly safely, provided the exercise is carefully prescribed and that the form and intensity of the activity are appropriate. Furthermore, the benefits of exercise are available to you, just as they are to those who don't have a history of heart disease – perhaps even more so. It is a good idea to talk to your doctor, specialist or cardiac nurse about the best way to increase your physical activity before you start.

*Note: The general advice about exercise given in this section applies whether you have a history of heart disease or not. Additional and more specific advice for those who have a history of heart problems is given later.*

# Action plan

Regular physical activity is essential to heart health, whether you already have a heart problem or not. If you would like to start a regular exercise programme, the remainder of this section will tell you how to go about it safely. If you are already taking regular physical exercise, it is still worth reading through the remainder of this section to check that you are on the right lines.

## How should I start?

The short answer is 'carefully'. *If you haven't exercised for a long time – and particularly if you are over 40 – it is very important to start gently and increase the amount of exercise you take gradually. If you are over 50, you would be wise to see your doctor before starting.* If you try to do too much too quickly, you risk getting injured and you may feel less inclined to exercise in the future. Ask yourself the following questions:

- Have you ever been told that you have a heart problem and advised to limit your physical activity?
- Do you have chest pain or discomfort which is brought on by exercise, e.g. when walking up a hill?
- Do you have episodes of dizziness or feeling faint?
- Are you a diabetic?
- Do you have any bone or joint problems that may limit, or be aggravated by, physical activity?
- Are you currently taking any medication for high blood pressure, angina or any other heart condition?
- Are you aware of any other health problem which may expose you to unnecessary risk during exercise?

If the answer to any of the above is 'Yes', then you should seek advice from your doctor before going any further.

And now a word about proper footwear and clothing. It is important that you use the correct tools for the job, otherwise you will be uncomfortable and increase the risk of injury. Walking or jogging on hard surfaces can be quite hard on the joints, so do invest in some sensible footwear. The technology involved in producing modern exercise footwear is remarkable – take full advantage of it. That old pair of flat shoes you found in the attic just will not do! So far as clothing is concerned, you can choose whatever you like – and the choice is fantastic. The only caveat is that functionality must still take precedence over fashion. It must be comfortable, cool in summer, warm in winter and allow a full range of movement.

## Getting started: Three questions

There are three questions to consider when preparing to exercise:

- Which exercise?
- How often (frequency) and how long (duration) should you exercise?
- How hard should the exercise be (intensity)?

## Which exercise?

The type of activity that benefits the cardio-respiratory system (the heart and lungs) is called 'aerobic'. Aerobic activity is any regular, rhythmic exercise involving large muscle groups, typical examples being brisk walking, swimming and cycling. A list of activities beneficial to the heart is given below in Table 9. Choose something from Group A which you enjoy and are, therefore, likely to comply with. Activities listed under Group B may be enjoyable, but are unlikely to be of very much benefit to your heart.

Apart from improving aerobic fitness, exercise may also improve strength, flexibility (suppleness) and muscular endurance. No singular exercise is 'pure' – all have several elements. But if a healthy heart is your goal, concentrate first on improving your aerobic capacity. You may want to add other forms of exercise, including light weight-training, later.

*Table 9*  Activities for a Healthy Heart

| *Group A – Good/Excellent* | *Group B – Poor* |
| --- | --- |
| Brisk walking | Yoga |
| Swimming | Golf |
| Cycling | Housework |
| Jogging/running | Light gardening |
| Badminton/tennis | Bowling |
| Gym-work (aerobics, stepping, treadmill, exercise bike etc) | Table-tennis |
| Hill-walking | Archery |
| Dancing | Darts |
| Ice skating | Horse riding |
| Hockey | |
| Netball | |

If you are significantly overweight, you would be well advised to choose non-weight bearing forms of activity such as stationary exercise bicycling or swimming. These will improve your fitness and help to get your weight down, whilst avoiding damage to joints and tendons. When your body weight has been reduced to more acceptable levels, you can safely add other activities such as brisk walking and badminton to your routine.

Here are some brief comments about the various forms of aerobic activity mentioned above.

**Walking** is the most natural of all exercises and has been undervalued in terms of its health-promoting properties. Indeed, evidence suggests that a *brisk* walk every day may offer health benefits comparable to those normally associated with more vigorous exercise. One recent study found that women who walk briskly (three to four miles per hour) for at least three hours per week can reduce their risk of heart attack and stroke by 54 per cent. All in all, brisk walking is a great exercise and one accessible to almost everyone – including the elderly and patients with heart disease. Examples of walking programmes are given in Appendix 4, p.241.

**Swimming** is an excellent exercise for improving fitness, but it also scores well for strength and flexibility. If I had to select one activity for everyone, it would be this one. Because your body weight is supported by the water, swimming is ideal for anyone with back or joint problems, or who is overweight. The obvious disadvantage is that you need to have ready access to a swimming pool. Even if this is geographically convenient, there may be other limitations. Pools are often crowded with children, especially during school holidays and at weekends. This may make steady, good-quality swimming hazardous or impossible. However, most pools have adult sessions at specific times, and if you choose your times carefully you should be able to establish a regular routine. It shouldn't cost much either – most pools now have season tickets and special rates for lunch-time or early morning sessions.

**Cycling (outdoors)** is a great exercise for cardiovascular fitness and, to a lesser extent, strength. It will do little for your flexibility, however, so you should add some stretching/flexibility exercises to your programme. There are few forms of exercise so enjoyable when the sun is shining and the leafy lanes beckon. The problem nowadays is that the roads are so congested with cars and heavy lorries, that cycling has become quite a dangerous form of recreation. It is also much more hazardous during the winter months when visibility is poor and the roads may be icy. I suggest sticking to cycling in the summer months and switching to other activities during winter.

If you're worried about the roads, stationary cycling using an exercise bike is an excellent alternative. It has the great benefit of being very convenient and, when used properly, is extremely effective. As a non-weight-bearing exercise it may also have particular advantages for those with joint or weight problems. Unfortunately, most people find it terminally boring – even with modern computer graphics which are meant to convince you that you're riding through the mountains of Colorado. But if you enjoy it – great! Some examples of cycling programmes are given in Appendix 4, p.243.

One last word here, *always* wear a crash helmet. The technology has improved enormously and nowadays the helmets are so light and well-ventilated that there really cannot be any excuse for not wearing one.

**Exercise machines** in health clubs, gyms or at home, are used by millions of people. The most popular examples are the treadmill, the cycle-ergometer (stationary bike), rowing machine, cross-country skier, and the stair stepper. The makers of these machines all claim superiority, but is there any real difference? A recent study suggests that the treadmill is the most effective indoor exercise machine, followed by the stair stepper, rowing ergometer, cross-country skier and stationary exercise bike. But the important thing is to buy what you find most suitable to you. Correctly used they are all excellent for the heart – and easy to get in front of the TV!

**Jogging and running** are still very popular, although much more so among men than women. Jogging improves cardio-respiratory fitness, but does much less for strength and flexibility. What exactly constitutes jogging as opposed to running is difficult to say, although it's usually taken that jogging is slower and less vigorous. Few people would argue that if you can cover a mile in six minutes or under you are running. If you take 10 or 20 minutes, you're jogging. At what point the one merges into the other is anyone's guess.

You can run almost anywhere, and although you run the risk of injury to feet, ankles and knees, wearing proper footwear can reduce this to a minimum. When running on pavements look out for pot-holes and also for low-level branches from trees and shrubs – they can inflict serious eye damage. Some examples of jogging programmes are given in Appendix 4, p.242.

### Frequency and duration

Having selected your exercise, you now have to consider how often and how long you should exercise to achieve a health benefit for your heart. The most authoritative guidelines are those from the US National Institutes of Health (1996), which state that:

> 'Children and adults alike, should set a goal of accumulating at least 30 minutes of moderate-intensity physical activity on most – and preferably all – days of the week.'

This means that if you cannot manage to do all your exercise at once, you can do it in smaller chunks throughout the day. For example, a brisk 15-minute walk to work in the morning and then again in the evening, means you have accumulated 30 minutes of moderately intensive activity. But what do we mean by *moderate* intensity?

## Intensity

How hard should the exercise be? There are two ways of assessing this: the Talk Test and the Training Heart Rate.

The simplest way is to use the **Talk Test**, which uses your ability to hold a conversation with someone as a measure of your exercise intensity. There are three levels:

*Level 1*: If you can hold a conversation with someone quite easily, without feeling at all out of breath, you are not working hard enough. Try harder!

*Level 2*: If you can hold a conversation, but feel a bit breathless, this is the correct intensity. Keep it up!

*Level 3*: If you find it very difficult to speak at all, you are working too hard. Ease up!

So, whatever physical activity you choose, Level 2 is where you should be. Moreover, you should feel pretty much back to normal within 10 minutes of stopping exercise and, if you don't, you are pushing yourself too hard.

The slightly more involved, but most accurate, indicator of exercise intensity is your **Training Heart Rate**, or pulse rate, expressed in beats per minute (beats/min). Everyone has a maximum heart rate that is related to his or her age, known as the Age Predicted Maximum Heart Rate (APMHR). This is simply the fastest your heart can beat. A simple way to calculate your APMHR is to subtract your age from 220, i.e:

$$APMHR = 220–Age \text{ (in years)}$$

So, if you are 50 years old, your APMHR is 220–50 = 170 beats/minute. This means that however hard you exercise, your heart will not beat any faster than 170 beats/min.

But how does this help in determining exercise intensity? Scientific studies have shown that the intensity of effort required for effective aerobic training is in the range of 60–75 per cent of the APMHR. This 60–75 per cent heart rate range is called the Training Zone. Training Zone heart rates for different age groups are shown in Table 10 opposite.

As you can see, if you are 40 years old, your Training Zone is between 108–135 beats per minute. When you begin your exercise programme,

*Table 10*  Training Zone heart rates

| Age (years) | Training Zone heart rate (60-75% of APMHR) | APMHR (220-age) |
|---|---|---|
| 20 | 120–150 beats/min | 200 |
| 25 | 117–146 beats/min | 195 |
| 30 | 114–142 beats/min | 190 |
| 35 | 111–139 beats/min | 185 |
| 40 | 108–135 beats/min | 180 |
| 45 | 105–131 beats/min | 175 |
| 50 | 102–127 beats/min | 170 |
| 55 | 99–124 beats/min | 165 |
| 60 | 96–120 beats/min | 160 |
| 65 | 93–116 beats/min | 155 |
| 70 | 90–113 beats/min | 150 |
| 75 | 87–109 beats/min | 145 |

aim for the lower end of your Training Zone heart rate (60 per cent) during the first couple of months. As your fitness improves you can gradually work up towards the upper limit (75 per cent). After six months, you can exercise above this level – as high as 80–85 per cent of your APMHR if you wish, but you don't have to work that hard to stay in good condition.

Since you are using heart rate (or pulse rate) to measure exercise intensity, you obviously need to be able to take your pulse accurately – a procedure which requires a little practice (see Taking Your Pulse, p.144). After a while, you will become quite good at estimating your heart rate without having to take it.

Nowadays, an even easier option to monitor your heart rate is to purchase an electronic pulse monitor. These are an excellent investment and allow you to monitor your own heart rate very accurately. A special belt is worn around the chest (this is not uncomfortable), which picks up the electrical signal from your heart. This signal is then sent to a wristwatch which has a large display, making it easy for you to see what's happening at any point during your exercise period. Any good-quality sports shop will stock a range of pulse monitors, but you don't need the most expensive model in town. Keep it as simple as possible.

## TAKING YOUR OWN PULSE

The pulse is the wave of pressure that passes along each artery following each beat of the heart. There are two places to take your own pulse: over the radial artery at the wrist and over the carotid artery in the neck. To take the radial pulse hold one hand palm upwards and place the pads of the three finger tips of the other hand on the groove on the outer side of the wrist – just above the wrist creases – in line with your thumb. You can feel the pulse quite clearly when your fingers are in the right place (Figure 23a).

Most people find it easier to take the carotid pulse during exercise. To do this, first feel your Adam's apple, then move your fingers about one-and-a-half inches either side of this and you will feel the carotid pulse (Figure 23b). *Never compress both carotid pulses at once.*

Using a watch with a second hand count the number of beats you can feel over 10 seconds, and multiply by six. So if you can feel 20 beats, your heart rate is 120 beats per minute. Alternatively, you can count over 15 seconds and multiply by four. Even easier, buy a pulse monitor!

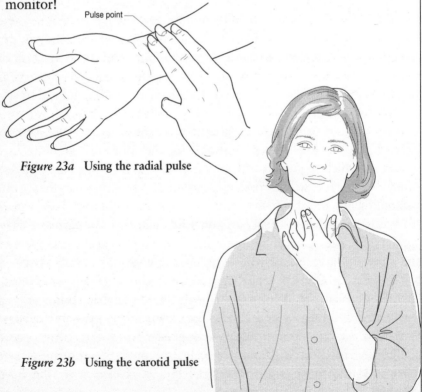

Pulse point

*Figure 23a*    Using the radial pulse

*Figure 23b*    Using the carotid pulse

## Warming up and cooling down

Whatever time of day you choose, always warm up gradually and cool down properly. Never exercise on a full stomach or after consuming alcohol. Gentle stretching of the limbs and muscles prior to exercising is good practice, and will reduce the likelihood of muscular strains during the exercise session proper. Drink small amounts of fluid frequently (every 10 minutes or so) during exercise. If you wait until you feel thirsty it's too late, you will already be dehydrated.

Cooling down is equally important. Never stop suddenly – take a few minutes to cool down to allow your system to return to normal. So, if you are walking briskly, slow down for a few minutes before stopping completely.

Finally, listen to what your body is telling you – if it doesn't feel right, *don't do it.*

## What about joining a gym or health club?

Few of us have the discipline to exercise alone, so joining a health club or gymnasium has obvious advantages. You can go along with your partner or a friend and make it a social occasion, and you don't have to worry about the weather. If you can get to the club at off-peak times, the membership fees are usually very reasonable. Most of the larger health club groups have trained physical instructors who will show you how to use equipment and design a personal exercise programme to suit your needs.

*If you have a heart condition you must let the club know at the time of joining.* They will normally ask you to obtain a letter from your doctor confirming that it's OK for you to start exercising.

## What about weight training?

Although many older people are aware of the importance of regular aerobic exercise such as walking or swimming, many tend to dismiss weight training (also called resistance training) as an activity for the young or the vain. In general, as we grow older, our muscle fibres atrophy (shrink in number and size) and become less sensitive to messages from the brain. This results in a decrease in strength, balance and coordination.

However, it is now clear that resistance training can substantially slow down and even reverse, the decline in muscle mass, bone density and strength that were once considered to be the inevitable consequences of ageing. Many patients with heart problems, including those who have had surgery, lack the physical strength and/or self-confidence to perform common activities of daily living. Mild to moderate resistance training improves muscular endurance and coordination, reduces coronary risk factors and leads to a greater sense of well-being. For those who have had CABG, graded resistance training – beginning when the wound has fully healed – can help restore normal muscle function in the chest and arms and restore normal posture.

In general, therefore, light to moderate weight training is strongly recommended as a complement to the usual aerobic activities described above. However, it is essential that you have proper instruction in the use of weights or resistance machines; overuse or inappropriate use can cause injury. Joining a good health club or gym is easily the best option, since expert guidance is readily available. Make sure you tell the fitness instructor about any heart problems and get the all-clear from your doctor before you begin.

Some general tips of resistance training:

- Speak to your doctor before you begin a resistance training programme.
- Make sure you have a reasonable standard of aerobic fitness before you start.
- Aim for 20–30 minutes of weight training two to three times per week.
- Use very light weights to begin with and aim for 12 to 15 repetitions per set of each exercise.
- Perform each movement slowly through the full range of motion that's possible for you.
- Focus on the large muscle groups, i.e. the legs, arms and chest.
- If you feel unwell at any time – STOP IMMEDIATELY.

## Physical activity for cardiac patients

The general advice about exercise above also applies to those with a history of heart problems. The target here, as for others, is to accumulate a minimum of 30 minutes' activity on most days of the week. There are, however, some additional general points to bear in mind.

Firstly, there is the question of the type of activity to be taken. Activities recommended for the heart are aerobic – i.e. they involve major muscle groups in a rhythmical fashion (e.g. brisk walking, swimming, cycling etc). But *isometric* exercise is quite different. An example of isometric exercise in everyday life is when you try to raise a jammed window, or lift an extremely heavy suitcase. This type of activity produces a sharp rise in blood pressure and puts a considerable strain on the heart muscle. If the heart is already damaged from a previous heart attack, or if you have high blood pressure, then activities such as lifting heavy objects, shovelling snow, heavy digging, etc. can be dangerous. If you have had heart surgery, isometric exercise can be painful and may cause movement in the chest wound. So for all patients with heart problems the advice is the same; *if there are heavy weights to be lifted, get someone else to do it!*

The second consideration is the intensity of the activity. The general advice is to start slowly with walking programmes (see below) and then move on to normal activities. Use the Talk Test to gauge the intensity of your exercise. If you use a Training Zone Heart Rate (see p.143), keep to the lower level initially and do not exceed the upper level heart rate. Consider investing in an electronic heart rate monitor.

Here are some general points for all heart patients:

- Start gradually and concentrate on aerobic activities such as walking on a treadmill, swimming or using a stationary exercise bicycle.
- Do not lift heavy weights (very light weight training may be beneficial later).
- If you feel unwell, or experience chest discomfort, palpitations or dizziness, stop exercising immediately.
- If you exercise with a partner, make sure they keep to your pace, not you to theirs.
- If you're playing a competitive game such as tennis or badminton, the rule is to always play well within *your* limits, not those of your partner/opponent.
- Do not exercise with a fever.
- Listen to what your body tells you and learn to distinguish the difference between genuinely not feeling well enough to exercise and being lazy. If you really don't feel like it – DON'T GO.

*If you are recovering from a heart attack or heart surgery:* General advice regarding the immediate period following a heart attack is given in Chapter 6. For the first four to six weeks following a heart attack, you should only carry out normal activities of daily living. At the end of that time you may join a cardiac rehabilitation programme, or you may start self-rehabilitation at home. To begin with, I suggest the following preliminary eight-week walking programme, which has been designed by the Toronto Cardiac Rehabilitation Centre:

*Level 1*:  For two weeks walk 1.6Km (1 mile) in 30 minutes
*Level 2*:  For two weeks walk 2Km (1$^1$/2 miles) in 42 minutes
*Level 3*:  For two weeks walk 3Km (2 miles) in 50 minutes
*Level 4*:  For two weeks walk 3.8Km (2$^1$/2 miles) in 57$^1$/2 minutes

*Note*: Walk on five days per week.

When you have completed this preliminary stage, I would suggest you move on to a more vigorous 12-week walking programme (See Appendix 4, p.241), beginning at the lowest level. After this you can then progress to a normal exercise programme, paying attention to type, frequency, duration and intensity. But to begin with, you should again start at the lower end of your Training Zone heart rate.

So, to summarise how to progress with physical activity patterns after discharge from hospital after a heart attack or after surgery:

---

### ACTIVITY TIME-SCALES FOLLOWING HEART ATTACK OR SURGERY

| *Period* | *Activities* |
| --- | --- |
| First 4–6 weeks | Normal activities of daily living: no structured exercise programme |
| Next 8 weeks | Preliminary walking programme |
| Next 12 weeks | Standard 12-week walking programme (see Appendix 4) |
| After the above | Normal activities – based on appropriate exercise prescription |

---

*If you have angina:* Again, a sensible starting point is the preliminary walking programme, progressing to a normal walking programme and beyond. Always stay within the limits of your angina. If you experience pain, stop and rest before continuing. Using nitroglycerine tablets or spray before you start to exercise will help.

*If you have hypertension:* Check with your doctor that your blood pressure is adequately controlled before you start to exercise. Start gently, monitor your blood pressure regularly and avoid activities which have a large isometric component (i.e. lifting heavy objects).

Note: *Some drugs used to treat angina and hypertension, such as beta-blockers, may interfere with the normal heart rate response, making it difficult to use the Training Zone heart rate to determine exercise intensity. Discuss this with your doctor, or use Level 2 of the Talk Test as a guide instead.*

## Checklist: Your exercise prescription

Having considered the type, frequency, duration and intensity for your exercise programme, the requirements for safe, effective exercise are summarized in the Exercise Prescription below. Armed with these simple principles, you can now go ahead and exercise effectively and safely, whether you already have heart problems or not.

---

### EXERCISE PRESCRIPTION

**Type**      Regular, rhythmical and involving major muscle groups
            – e.g. brisk walking, swimming, cycling

**Frequency**   Most days of the week

**Duration**   At least 30 minutes accumulated during the day

**Intensity**   At moderate intensity (Talk Test Level 2)

            60–75 per cent of your Age Predicted Maximum Heart
            Rate

Notes:
- Patients recovering from a heart attack should begin with a preliminary walking programme
- Those with other heart problems or who are very unfit, should start with either a preliminary or the standard walking programme
- After completing the walking programmes, progress freely to other aerobic activities of your choice – i.e. swimming, cycling
- During exercise, keep to Level 2 of the Talk Test or within the appropriate Training Zone heart rate for your age
- Consider adding light weight training under expert supervision

---

# Action File 5

# Achieving a healthier weight

Carrying too much weight puts an extra strain on your heart and greatly increases your risk of a range of other diseases, including arthritis, diabetes, respiratory problems and some forms of cancer. If you already have evidence of heart trouble, it is all the more important to achieve and maintain a healthier weight. Modern society encourages us to eat more and to be less active, which explains why most of us have a tendency to gain weight if we are not careful. The key to successful weight loss is to understand the energy equation. By reducing energy (food) intake, and increasing energy expenditure (physical activity), you can restore your energy equation to a healthy balance. You should adopt a low-fat, but nutritionally balanced diet and combine this with a regular programme of moderate physical activity. Learn how to eat smart, shop smart and cook smart and moderate your alcohol intake. Aim to get your waist measurement down to a safe level by losing one to two pounds of fat weight per week, and aim for a *healthier* weight, rather than your cosmetic ideal. Put your heart health first!

## Background

Despite the exhortations of various health professionals to eat less and exercise more, the national waistline continues to expand at an alarming rate. Millions of Britons, along with the populations of most industrialised countries, have been getting fatter for years. During the past two decades the proportion of those who are overweight has risen by 50 per cent and obesity has nearly trebled. The latest figures show that more than half the adult population is overweight, and about one in five is obese (21 per cent of women and 17 per cent of men). This means that in all likelihood one out of two of you reading this, is technically overweight or obese. Moreover, crude projections suggest that by the year 2025, levels of obesity in this country could be as high as 30–40 per cent and

45–50 per cent in the USA. The irony is that we are getting fatter at a time when multi-billion pound markets in diet programmes, low-fat foods, health clubs and other slimming aids are booming.

## Energy balance

To understand why we put on weight, or lose it, you first need to understand the concept of energy balance. Most women are familiar with counting calories (or joules, which is the metric term for calories). A calorie is the unit used to describe the energy content of food and drink, as well as the energy we use in the normal physical activities of living. The energy equation states that the energy we take in from food and drink, minus the energy we expend through exercise and other activities of daily living, determines whether our energy balance is positive, neutral or negative i.e:

**Energy Intake – Energy Expenditure = Energy Balance**

Here are three examples to illustrate the point:

### Example 1: Weight gain

A woman has a daily energy intake of 2500 calories and an energy expenditure of 2000; in other words, she is taking in 500 calories more than she expends, so she will gain weight. We say that she is in *positive energy balance* – the excess energy is stored as fat. Her energy equation is:

| 2500 | – | 2000 | = | Positive Energy Balance ( +500) |

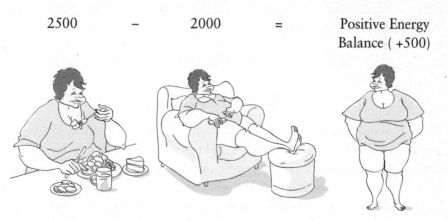

### Example 2: Weight constant

Here a woman has a daily energy intake of 2000 and an energy expenditure of 2000; in other words she is taking in precisely the same number of calories as she expends – so her weight will not change. Here we say that the energy equation is *balanced* or *neutral*, i.e:

2000          –          2000          =          Neutral Energy
                                                  Balance (0)

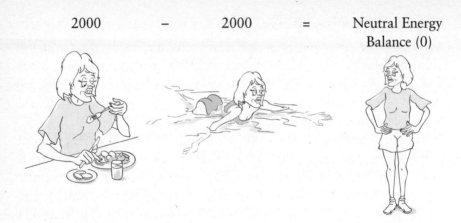

## Example 3: Weight loss

In the last example, a woman has a daily energy intake of 2000 calories and an energy expenditure of 2500; this means that she takes in fewer calories than she needs – so she will lose weight. We say that she is in *negative energy balance*, i.e:

2000          –          2500          =          Negative Energy
                                                  Balance (–500)

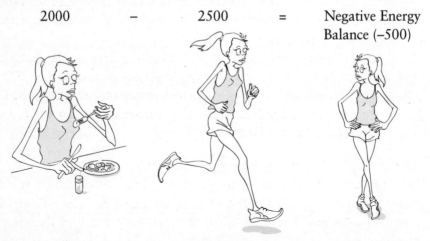

Nature provided primitive man with this beautifully balanced mechanism, by means of which energy intake and expenditure could be balanced and body weight remain relatively stable. Most of the energy from food eaten by early man was used quickly, but the ability to store a certain amount as fat conferred a strong survival advantage and acted as a buttress against harder times when food was scarce. (*Note*: It is an incredibly efficient mechanism – 500g (1lb) of fat stores 3500 calories.) In addition, hunting and gathering food involved high levels of physical activity – and hence energy expenditure – which helped keep the energy equation balanced.

## Why are we getting fatter?

In modern society, the natural and healthy balance of our ancestors has been profoundly changed. The wide availability of energy-dense foods and larger portions, etc, combined with the fact that we are less active than ever, has resulted in the energy equation being strongly weighted towards positive energy balance.

The situation is made more difficult because society gives us powerful but conflicting messages. On the one hand we are told that to be thin is to be attractive, desirable and successful; on the other we are constantly exposed to seductive images of delicious, fattening, easily available and inexpensive food. The explosion of TV programmes about food and cooking and the amount of space bookstores now devote to cookery and recipe books, are testimony to the growing national obsession with food. Eating is no longer simply a means of acquiring the necessary energy and nutrients for living; for many people it has become a fully fledged leisure-time activity. Moreover, a good deal of our diet has become based around fast foods; Britain consumes more pizza, burgers and chips than any other country in Europe. So it might seem obvious that we are getting fatter because we are eating more. But is this true?

You may be surprised to know that average energy intake (calories from food) in Britain has *fallen* by around 20 per cent since the 1970s. This is why many doctors and scientists believe that the most likely explanation for the obesity epidemic is not that we are eating too much, but that we are exercising too little.

## Your energy equation – the key to weight control

Obesity, then, can be regarded as a chronic energy imbalance, in which intake exceeds expenditure and the excess energy is stored as fat. If your intake exceeds your output by 500 calories per day, in the course of one week you will put on 500g (1lb) of fat (since 500g of fat is equivalent to 3500 calories). But often the daily energy excess is not very great. For example, even if your intake exceeds your expenditure by just 50 calories a day (the equivalent of one digestive biscuit) you will put on 2.2Kg (5lb) of fat weight each year – and 11Kg (25lb) in five years. It is a *small* excess over a *long* period that does the damage.

Although many people with weight problems find the energy equation easy to understand, they seem to think that in their case it doesn't quite apply. They argue that they don't eat as much as other people and yet they continue to gain weight. How can we explain why it is that some people have this tendency to put on weight, while others seem to be able to eat anything they want and never put on an ounce (we all know them)? Let's deal firstly with the myths and then with the facts.

## Glands and 'thrifty metabolism' – the myths about weight gain

Many people think that their weight problems are due to 'glandular problems'. It's true that there are some medical conditions which result in weight gain, e.g. an underactive thyroid gland, but these are uncommon causes of weight gain.

A more common misconception is that some people have a thrifty metabolism – i.e. a low metabolic rate, which means they don't burn as much energy as the next person and, therefore, gain weight. This is also completely incorrect. In fact, their Resting Metabolic Rate (RMR) is *higher* than that of thin people as the heart, liver and other vital organs are bigger and need more energy to function (see p.165). For example, a 40-year-old woman weighing 60Kg (133lb) will have an RMR of about 1340 calories per day, whereas a 100Kg (217lb) woman will need 1660 calories (an extra 24 per cent) just to maintain her weight and normal functions.

## So why do some people gain weight and not others?

Given that most of us are prone to put on weight in the right circumstances, which factors make some of us more susceptible than others?

### Genetics

It is clear that obesity runs in families. Children with two obese parents have about a 70 per cent risk of becoming obese, compared with less than 20 per cent in children of lean parents. This might be explained by environmental factors, since families usually share the same diet, lifestyle and cultural influences. However, studies of adopted children show weight patterns which are closer to those of their natural (biological) parents than their adopted parents, suggesting that there is a strong genetic contribution to weight problems. It is not easy to say how much genetic factors contribute in any individual case – it may be anywhere from five per cent to more than 50 per cent. Genes may exert their effects by increasing energy intake or decreasing energy expenditure, for example through a genetically determined preference for high fat foods or a sedentary lifestyle. They may also influence appetite regulation. However, the rapid increase in obesity during the past 50 years suggests that obesity is more strongly determined by diet and activity patterns than by genes, since the 'gene pool' in the general population would not have changed so dramatically during such a short period of time.

### Ethnicity

There are marked ethnic differences in the likelihood of obesity, with Black and Hispanic groups at much greater risk than Caucasians. Important differences also exist in fat distribution. Asian immigrants in the UK have more central (abdominal) fat than native Caucasians and in Europe, Mediterranean women have more central fat than Northern European women. These differences are likely to be due to a combination of genetic, cultural and social factors.

### Social class

In developed countries, the proportion of those with weight problems is higher in lower social classes than in more affluent groups. Although there are many theories to explain why this might be, none is entirely satisfactory.

### Medical disorders and drugs

As we saw above, a very few individuals have underlying medical conditions which lead to obesity. Patients with these conditions (for example, hypothyroidism and Cushing's syndrome) are usually identified quickly by their symptoms and their overall physical appearance.

Certain drugs, such as steroids (used to treat asthma and arthritis), can also promote fat storage in certain parts of the body. Some antihistamines and antidepressants may also result in weight gain, although this usually reverses when the treatment ends.

### Psychological factors

People respond differently to stressful life events. Some tend to eat less, but for many others the phenomenon of 'comfort eating' can lead to excessive weight gain. There is also considerable variation in the level of control individuals are able to exert over their environment. Clearly some people find it much easier to control energy (food) intake than others.

So the tendency for any one individual to put on weight will depend upon a combination of factors, including genetics, ethnicity, cultural background, medical history, medication and psychological make-up. But please understand that this does not alter the fundamental cause of obesity, namely that energy (food) intake exceeds energy expenditure. These factors simply help to explain why some people tend to put on weight more easily than others. The key point is that we each have our own energy equation. If we are lucky, we can eat to our heart's content and never put on an ounce. For most of us, however, our energy equation isn't quite so kind. Effective weight management is all about learning how to manage your own unique energy equation.

## Weight gain during pregnancy

Records from obesity clinics show that 50–80 per cent of female patients blame pregnancy for their weight problems. Recent studies show:

- Women who gain more than 16 kg (35lb) during pregnancy are likely to remain 4–9Kg (10–20lbs) heavier than their pre-pregnant weight 12 months after giving birth.
- Women who have more children are likely to be heavier during pregnancy than those with fewer children.
- About half the body fat gained during pregnancy is deposited as the high-risk abdominal (or central) fat – see p.158.
- Overweight and obese women are more likely to develop diabetes brought on by their pregnancy and this increases the risk of diabetes and heart disease in later life.
- Excessive weight gain during pregnancy not only puts the mother at increased risk of remaining overweight or obese, but is likely to complicate future pregnancies.

Modest weight gain during pregnancy is essential, but continuing to gain weight after the birth of the baby is neither desirable nor inevitable. Of course, the demands of a new baby, together with changes in dietary and lifestyle habits, can make weight loss in the months following the birth very difficult. Nevertheless, it is important to begin the process of returning to the pre-pregnancy weight, even if the goal for the first couple of months is simply to avoid any further weight increase.

## Weight gain during menopause

The hormonal changes which occur at the time of the menopause lead to significant changes in fat distribution. Fat begins to accumulate around the waist, rather than the hips and thighs, leading to 'central' obesity instead of the usual pear-shape of younger women. This has important health implications (see p.157). Although many women complain that maintaining a healthy weight is more difficult at this time than any other, there is no physiological reason why this should be the case. The most likely explanation is that women become much less physically active as they get older, but maintain or increase their food intake. Some women also blame HRT for their weight gain, but again there is no physiological basis for such an association. It's all down to the energy equation I'm afraid.

## The health consequences of obesity

The fact that people are getting bigger is not, in itself, cause for concern – after all, we could just make things bigger to accommodate them.

Boeing's aeroplane designers now build seats designed to take passengers who are 9Kg (20lb) heavier than they were since their first airliners took to the skies. Designers of clothes, furniture, beds, and cars also acknowledge that customers are getting larger. But the real reason why we should be concerned is that obesity has a variety of important *health* consequences, including:

- Heart and circulatory diseases (see below).
- Varicose veins.
- Cancer (particularly breast cancer in women).
- Gallstones.
- Arthritis and degenerative joint disease.
- Back pain.
- Respiratory (lung) disease.
- Sleep apnoea (a potentially dangerous condition in which the individual snores heavily and may actually stop breathing for long periods).
- Depression and low self-esteem.

## Apples, pears and heart disease

As we saw in Chapter 3, obesity increases heart risks mainly through its association with other CHD risk factors such as hypertension and abnormal blood lipids. But why do these factors cluster together in the first place? It turns out that the real culprit in all this is *insulin*.

The problem with being overweight is not simply the fat itself, but *where* it is deposited. Women who are 'pear shaped' – with fat distributed over their hips and thighs – seem to be at much lower risk of heart disease than those who are 'apple shaped', i.e. with fat carried around the abdomen, particularly at the front, like the typical beer belly in men (see Figure 27). To put it bluntly, a pot belly is bad news. This is because when fat cells are deposited over the abdomen, they seem to make the body more resistant to the effects of insulin. Individuals who are insulin resistant compensate by producing higher blood levels of insulin than normal and, in some cases, become overtly diabetic.

Raised insulin levels also increase blood pressure, cholesterol and triglycerides, lower HDL-C and increase the tendency for the blood to form clots – all of which contribute to a greater risk of heart attack and stroke. Insulin is, therefore, the single factor which connects obesity with a variety of risk factors associated with an increased risk of heart disease (see Figure 28). This 'clustering' together of risk factors has been given a special name, Insulin Resistance Syndrome (IRS). Women who have central (abdominal) obesity and IRS have a greatly increased risk of heart attack.

*Figure 27*  Patterns of obesity

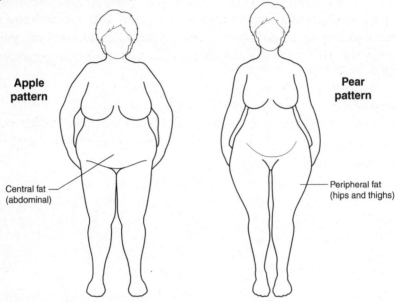

*Figure 28*  The Insulin Resistance Syndrome (IRS)

*Note.* Abdominal fat leads to insulin resistance and the various components of IRS, which leads to increased risk of cardiovascular disease.

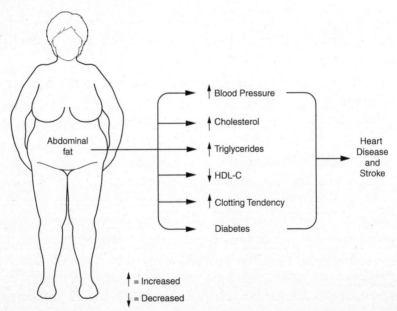

## Measuring obesity – are you at risk?

There are several ways to measure obesity:

**Charts.** Most of you will be familiar with the charts in magazines and books which are supposed to tell you what your desirable weight is, based on height, weight and frame size. Most of these charts are based on tables originally developed by the Metropolitan Life Insurance company, but they are poor indicators of health risks and are no longer recommended.

**Body Mass Index (BMI).** This commonly used system is a measure of your weight relative to your height. BMI is calculated by taking your weight in kilograms and dividing this by the square of your height in metres i.e:

$$BMI = \frac{Weight\ (Kg)}{Height\ (m)^2}$$

Doctors commonly use BMI to classify an individual's weight as follows:

Less than 25   – Healthy
25–30              – Overweight
Over 30            – Obese

So, when doctors talk about patients who are obese, or the proportion of obese people in the population, they are referring to those with a BMI greater than $30Kg/m^2$.

**Waist measurement.** This is by far the simplest method, and the most accurate predictor of health risks. To measure your waist circumference properly, use a cloth tape and:

- Put the tape directly onto your waist – i.e. next to the skin *not* over clothing.
- Make sure the tape is at the level of the navel.
- Don't pull too tightly – let the tape fit snugly around your waist.
- Try to measure in the same place each time.

This is how waist circumference is related to health risks in women:

*Table 11*  Waist size and health risks in women

| Level 1 | Level 2 | Level 3 |
|---|---|---|
| Less than 80 cms (32 ins) | 80-88 cms (32-35 ins) | More than 88 cms (35 ins) |
| HEALTHY | INCREASED RISK | HIGH RISK |

Before moving on to the Action Plan proper, it is important to introduce the word 'health' at this point. Much of the writing about weight and slimming is based on the idea that fatness is unattractive. Because of this, the association between weight and health invariably plays second fiddle to the cosmetic benefits of weight loss. No harm in that you may say; the way people see themselves is important to promoting confidence and self-esteem. However, to encourage vulnerable individuals to lose weight in an effort to achieve an idealised image promoted by those whose only interest is in selling magazines, drugs, or weekends on 'fat farms', is both absurd and dangerous. This is not a trivial issue. Many overweight women are taking serious risks with extreme forms of dieting and drugs, when the 'goal' weight they are trying to attain is completely unrealistic and, very often, unnecessary.

My aim in this section is to encourage those of you who are overweight, to achieve a *healthier* weight – not necessarily one which is cosmetically ideal. Because waist circumference is so strongly related to health risks, it provides a simple and relevant measure for monitoring healthy weight loss.

# Action plan

To establish whether or not you need to lose weight, take your waist measurement as described on p.159; your weight goal will obviously depend upon your waist size.

**Level 1   Waist less than 80cms (32ins)**
Your current weight is not likely to be associated with significant health risks. Maintain your healthy weight by paying close attention to your diet and physical activity patterns.
   *Your Goal:* Maintaining current weight.

**Level 2   Waist 80–88cms (32–35ins)**
You are at an increased risk of heart disease and other health problems. If you already have heart disease you would do well to get your weight down; even modest degrees of overweight place an unacceptable burden on a damaged heart. Follow the action plan to achieve a healthier weight.
   *Your Goal:* A waist measurement in the 'healthy' range – i.e. less than 80cm (32in).

**Level 3   Waist more than 88cms (35ins)**
A waist circumference greater than 88cm (35in) suggests that you have a

good deal of central (abdominal) fat, and this places you in a high risk category, particularly if you already have a history of heart disease.

*Your Goal:* The immediate aim should be to reduce your waist measurement to less than 88cm (35in). Depending on your progress, and how large your waist circumference was to begin with, try to get it as close to 80cm (32in) as possible.

If your waist measurement is above 100cm (40in), aim to lose 10cms (4in) as a first action goal, and then reduce in a stepwise fashion until you are below 88cm (35in). If you can get below 80cm (32in) all well and good, but it is more important to maintain your weight at a realistic level than to make impossible demands upon yourself. Far better that you should keep your waist circumference in the Level 2 range of 80–88cm (32–35in), than to try and repeatedly fail to achieve and maintain Level 1.

Remember, any decrease in your waist measurement is progress.

## Sensible weight loss

Having set sensible goals, how do you actually achieve them? Let's first remind ourselves of where we started – the energy equation (see p.151).

The energy equation is a physical law of the universe – there are no exceptions! Although a variety of factors and life events may predispose an individual to become overweight, no one is inevitably condemned to be obese. Ultimately, overweight only develops when energy intake exceeds expenditure.

To lose weight, you need to create a state of negative energy balance. To do this, you will need to:

Reduce energy (food) intake
*or*
Increase energy output (physical activity)
*or*
Both

In practice, the sensible approach is to reduce energy intake and increase energy output.

*Remember: Your aim is to create a negative energy balance (or energy deficit) of around 500–600 calories per day, which means you will lose about 500–750g(1–1¹/₂lb) of fat weight each week.*

Let's consider reducing energy intake and increasing energy expenditure separately.

## Reducing energy intake

There are six main dietary strategies to reduce energy intake:

Strategy 1   Reduce your fat intake.
Strategy 2   Eat a balanced diet.
Strategy 3   Reduce alcohol.
Strategy 4   Eat smart.
Strategy 5   Shop smart.
Strategy 6   Cook smart.

### Strategy 1: Reduce your fat intake

Studies show that dietary fat consumption plays a key role in the development of weight problems. The proportion of fat in the UK diet has doubled since the Second World War, and there is evidence to show that overweight people tend to have diets which are higher in fat than the average. One of the reasons for this is that fat is a highly palatable substance and adds both texture and taste to food. It is also 'energy-dense' containing twice as many calories per gram as protein or carbohydrate (see Table 12).

*Table 12*   Food energy values (calories per gram)

| | |
|---|---|
| Carbohydrate | 4 calories |
| Protein | 4 calories |
| Alcohol | 7 calories |
| Fat | 9 calories |

But perhaps the most important factor is that dietary fat does not seem to promote the same 'stop eating' signals that a similar quantity of carbohydrate or protein would. The result is that more fat calories tend to be consumed to achieve the same feeling of fullness and satisfaction than with other food groups. Therefore, the most effective way to reduce calorie intake, is to reduce the fat content of your diet.

To reduce your fat – and calorie – consumption, follow a low-fat diet. The principles are the same as those for a cholesterol-lowering diet (see p.111).

## REDUCING YOUR FAT INTAKE

- Eat fish, poultry without the skin and leaner cuts of meat (trim the visible fat away)
- Eat fewer high-fat processed meats, such as sausage, meat pies, salami, luncheon meat and hot dogs
- Limit your consumption of cheese, cream, eggs and other dairy products which tend to be high in fat
- Drink less whole milk and substitute either semi-skimmed or skimmed milk (which are actually a richer source of calcium)
- Increase your consumption of fresh vegetables and fruit and try to eat a purely vegetarian meal once or twice a week
- Eat more cereals, bread, pasta and other wholegrain products
- Reduce your intake of chocolates, cakes, pastries and biscuits which tend to contain large amounts of fat
- Try to use the frying pan less often; grill, bake or boil instead. Microwave cooking is particularly helpful. If you do fry, then use a monounsaturated oil (e.g. olive oil, rapeseed oil) or a polyunsaturated oil (e.g. safflower oil, sunflower oil)
- Avoid creamy dressings or sauces – look for low-fat or oil-free dressings
- When shopping, read the food labels and choose products with less than 5g fat per 100 g of food

### Strategy 2: Eat a balanced diet

When you are trying to lose weight, you must not only reduce your intake of saturated fat, as shown above, but you must also eat a good variety of foods to ensure you get the range of nutrients your body needs. Follow the 'Balance of Good Health' guidelines in Part III, p.222.

### Strategy 3: Reduce alcohol

As we saw earlier, alcohol contains seven calories per gram, compared with nine calories for fat and only four for protein and carbohydrate. So, on a weight-for-weight basis, alcohol is the second richest source of calories. But the energy content of an alcoholic drink is not simply related to the alcohol content, since many drinks contain sugars, carbohydrates and even small amounts of fat. The calorific value of some drinks based on *average* pub measures is shown in Table 13.

*Table 13*   Alcohol calorie counts

| | | | |
|---|---|---|---|
| 1 glass red wine | 90 | 1 glass sherry | 70 |
| 1 glass white wine | 80 | 1 glass port | 80 |
| 1 glass champagne | 80 | 1 Margarita | 175 |
| 1 gin and tonic | 140 | half pint of lager | 80 |
| 1 vodka and orange | 130 | Bloody Mary | 170 |
| 1 whisky | 70 | | |

Alcohol also has the effect of stimulating the appetite and of inhibiting willpower. If you have had a couple of glasses of wine you are much more likely to say 'Oh blow the diet – I'll worry about it tomorrow'.

So, if you need to lose weight should you stop drinking entirely? Some argue that because alcohol only contributes about two to four per cent of most women's total daily calorie intake there isn't much point in depriving yourself of the odd glass of wine. My own view is that losing weight is difficult enough, so if the *occasional* glass of wine helps you feel a bit less deprived, it is probably not a bad idea (but note the emphasis on occasional).

**Strategy 4: Eat smart**
Here's how to get smart about eating – and get those pounds off!

- Don't starve yourself for long periods – eat three or four smaller meals spaced throughout the day.
- Eat a healthy breakfast every day – cereals, orange juice, fruit etc.
- Try not to eat on the run – you will tend to eat 'junk' foods which are laden with fat and calories.
- Drink a glass of water before you start a meal. This will help you feel full and eat less.
- Reduce your portion sizes, use a smaller plate.
- If you use margarine or butter on bread, scrape it on in a very thin layer.
- Get into the habit of refusing second helpings.
- Chew your food slowly – take time to eat and digest your food slowly.
- Clear away all food when the meal is over – this will stop you picking at left-overs.

**Strategy 5: Shop smart**
- Try not to shop when you are hungry.
- Learn to read food labels (see p.218) and choose foods which have no more than 5g of fat per 100g of food product.

- Use a shopping list and don't buy anything that isn't on it.
- Choose lower-fat alternatives – i.e. skimmed milk and low-fat salad dressings.
- Fill your shopping trolley with plenty of vegetables, fruits, grains (pasta, rice and cereals).
- Avoid buying too many ready-made meals as they can be very high in fat.

**Strategy 6: Cook smart**

- Choose the leanest cuts of meat and cut away all visible fat before cooking; always remove the skin from poultry.
- Cut down on cooking oil by using non-stick cookware.
- Try not to fry – bake, steam, grill, boil, microwave or stir-fry instead.
- Don't prepare more than you need.
- Use low-fat recipes – bookshops and libraries have an amazing range of low-fat cookbooks.
- Base the meal on vegetables, salads and grains (rice, pasta etc), rather than the meat component, and try to eat one or two purely vegetarian meals each week.
- Keep out of the kitchen – eat to live, not live to eat!

## Increasing energy expenditure

There are three components to daily energy expenditure (see Figure 30): resting metabolic rate (RMR), physical activity, and thermogenesis.

*Figure 30*  Daily energy expenditure

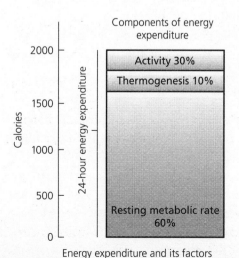

Energy expenditure and its factors

## Resting metabolic rate (RMR)

RMR is best thought of as the fuel used by a car when the engine is idling but the car isn't moving. It's the energy we use at rest, just to maintain our normal bodily functions such as breathing, digestion, etc, and it accounts for about 60 per cent of our daily energy expenditure.

## Physical activity

This includes all activities of daily living such as shopping, housework, walking and gardening etc, together with all leisure-time physical exercise (gym, badminton etc). It accounts for about 30 per cent of daily energy expenditure.

## Thermogenesis

Small additional amounts of energy are used for digestion, to keep us warm and to respond to stress – this is called thermogenesis. It accounts for about 10 per cent of energy expenditure.

Because it is difficult to change RMR or thermogenesis directly, the best way to increase energy expenditure is to increase your physical activity.

Action File 4, p.131, covers physical activity in detail, but the principles are:

- Start gently, and increase your physical activity gradually.
- If you are not already exercising, start with a walking programme.
- Aim to accumulate a minimum of 30 minutes' exercise each day.
- If you are carrying a lot of weight, or you have joint problems, begin with non-weight-bearing forms of activity, such as swimming or cycling on a stationary exercise bike.
- Try to be more active during your normal working day by using the stairs instead of the lift, getting off the bus or tube a couple of stops before home etc.
- Keep a diary of your activity patterns.

It is very difficult to lose weight by means of exercise or physical activity alone. Table 14 shows the average number of calories burned every hour for various activities. Given that 500g (1lb) of fat contains 3500 calories, you can see that you would need to walk at 4 m.p.h. for about nine hours to lose 500g (1lb) of fat. This observation is sometimes used by overweight people as an excuse for limiting their activity patterns and concentrating on diet alone as a means of losing weight.

*Table 14*   Physical activity and calories

**Burning calories**

| Activity | Calories/hour |
| --- | --- |
| Gardening | 165 |
| Housework (general) | 200 |
| Walking (3 mph) | 260 |
| Golf | 265 |
| Badminton | 360 |
| Walking (4 mph) | 400 |
| Cycling (10 mph) | 410 |
| Tennis (singles) | 450 |
| Cycling (13 mph) | 525 |
| Jogging (5 mph) | 550 |
| Swimming (continuous) | 650 |

But this view ignores two important points about physical activity.

Firstly, energy expenditure is cumulative. The way to look at it is not in terms of daily expenditure, but of monthly expenditure. Walking briskly for 30 minutes on five occasions per week, will amount to around 4000 calories per month – i.e. well over 500g (1lb) of fat weight. Longer periods of exercise will contribute even more.

Secondly – and most importantly – increasing physical activity is vital for weight maintenance and also helps to preserve valuable muscle tissue when people are losing weight. Precisely why exercise should be so effective in maintaining weight loss is not entirely clear, but evidence would suggest that it acts through a combination of mechanisms, including appetite suppression, reduced fat intake and preservation of lean body (muscle) mass. It's also clear that regular activity improves self-esteem and self-confidence which may further contribute to more effective weight maintenance (see Table 15).

*Table 15*   Mechanisms linking physical activity with effective weight maintenance

- Increased energy expenditure
- Better control of food intake    – reduced appetite
                                     – reduced fat consumption
- Improved body composition    – loss of fat
                                     – preservation of lean tissue
- Increased thermogenic response
- Increased insulin sensitivity
- Positive psychological effects

To conclude this section, here are some frequently asked questions about weight loss and weight maintenance.

### Should I count calories?

In the past, weight-management schemes have encouraged calorie-counting as a key part of successful weight loss, although there is no evidence that this is any more effective than simply reducing the fat content of your diet and becoming more physically active. Not only is calorie-counting tedious, it is also unnecessary. So my advice is that you should stop worrying about the specific calorie content of individual foods and focus on the *general* principles of weight loss, i.e. avoiding fat and increasing physical activity. Remember, there are no 'bad' foods – only bad diets.

### How much weight should I lose and how quickly?

Evidence shows that the most effective weight loss can be achieved from an energy deficit of 500–600 calories a day, which equates to a weight loss of around 500–750g (1–1¹/2lb) of fat weight per week. There is no benefit in trying to lose weight any faster than this, because you will be less likely to sustain it in the longer term. Clearly, if you have a lot of weight to lose, it may well take a long time to get to where you want to be, but you need to be patient. Take each day at a time, but think ahead; if you lose weight at the recommended rate, in three months you can lose 7–9Kg (15–20lb). Another simple guide to weight loss is the change in waist circumference; aim for a reduction of 5–10cm (2–4in) in two to three months.

### What should I eat if I feel hungry?

One of the hardest parts about trying to lose weight is feeling hungry much of the time. Choosing carbohydrates with a low Glycaemic Index (see p.212) will satisfy your hunger for longer, making it easier to control your food intake and lose weight. So, rather than rushing to eat crisps, biscuits, salted peanuts or other energy-dense foods, have some low-fat alternatives handy, e.g. oatmeal biscuits, low fat yogurt, apples, apricots (fresh and dried), pears, grapes, cherries, plums, kiwi fruit, All-Bran and Special K breakfast cereals.

### Eating out

Eating out a lot is not terribly good for losing weight. Because you have little control on what's available, you will inevitably have to compromise to some extent – and it's right that you should. After all, dining out is supposed to be relaxing and enjoyable; if you spend the whole time worrying about the food, you run the risk of becoming a diet bore. The important thing is to learn how to make smarter choices from the menu. It is bound to be a compromise to some extent but by selecting food options which have the lowest fat content you can limit the damage. Turn to Appendix 3, p.236, for some tips on eating out.

## Why don't 'crash diets' work?

Almost every week there will be some new dieting craze – a quick, painless and easy solution to your weight problem. It's quite true that crash dieting will allow you to lose weight very rapidly, particularly in the first week. The problem is that only a very small proportion of the weight lost will be fat – most of it is fluid. After losing weight, most people just go back to their old eating habits and the weight is rapidly regained. This type of crash dieting doesn't help people to learn how to adjust their eating habits to provide a diet which is sustainable in the longer term. Moreover, 'yo yo' dieting and weight loss is harmful to health, and can also lead to loss of confidence in the ability to lose weight in the long term.

The bottom line is that there are **NO QUICK FIXES – NONE!**

## How often should I weigh myself?

This is a very personal thing. Some women find regular feedback on their progress helpful and encouraging. Others despair at their lack of progress and become very discouraged at how much weight they still need to lose to get to their goal. Fluid changes alone can lead to quite marked fluctuations in weight, so remember that the scales are only a very general guide to progress – don't become a slave to them. Keep a record of your weight, and measure your waist circumference at regular intervals. As a general guide, I suggest you weigh yourself every week and take your waist measurement every two weeks. The exception to this is when you are trying to *maintain* your weight loss, when more frequent weighing is important.

## Should I keep a food and activity diary?

YES! Keeping track of what you are eating during the day is a great way to stay in control. Make sure you write it all down – including snacks – and take some time each week to see where you can improve. It's also a good idea to record your activity patterns in the same diary.

## What is successful weight loss?

Successful weight loss should be regarded in terms of a reduction in *health risks* – not merely the achievement of a particular body weight. This is why I have suggested using the waist measurement as your primary goal. We know that the larger the waist, the greater the likelihood of insulin resistance and the higher the risk of heart disease. Reducing your waist measurement will almost certainly reduce your health risks, as well as making you look and feel better. In fact, studies show that women who lose as little as 4–9Kg (10–20lb) can:

- Halve their risk of diabetes.
- Reduce both systolic and diastolic blood pressure by 10 mmHg.
- Reduce their cholesterol by 10 per cent and LDL-C by 15 per cent.
- Reduce their cancer risk by 40–50 per cent.

These are important health benefits which can be achieved by relatively modest weight loss. So don't worry if you are unable to reach what you – or others – may regard as a cosmetically ideal weight. It may be completely unrealistic to start with and repeated attempts to achieve it are likely to fail. Even if you succeed, you will probably be unable to maintain it. So the message is: be prepared to accept a weight that reduces your health risks and is maintainable, even if it doesn't correspond to your ideal.

## Why does it get more difficult to lose weight over time?

This is probably the most frequently asked question of all! The key to understanding why is to grasp the fact that as you weigh less, you need fewer calories to maintain your weight, so it becomes harder to create and sustain an energy deficit, i.e. negative energy balance. To illustrate my point, let's look at a typical pattern of weight loss over a period of several months in Figure 32.

At the beginning of the process, the person weighs W1 and needs 2000 calories to maintain that weight. She reduces her energy intake to 1400 calories, and so had an energy deficit of 600 calories per day, resulting in weight loss of about 750g (1½lb) a week for the first month.

At the end of month 1, she now weighs W2 – about 2.6Kg (6lb) less than W1, her initial weight. She stays on her 1400 calorie diet, but because she now weighs less than she did originally, she now needs only 1800 calories to maintain her new weight. This means that the energy deficit is less – 400 per day – so she will lose about 375g (¾lb) a week.

*Figure 32*  The pattern of weight loss

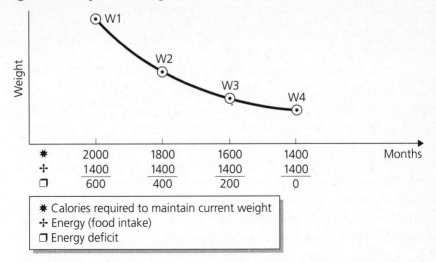

| ✳ | 2000 | 1800 | 1600 | 1400 | Months |
|---|------|------|------|------|--------|
| ✢ | 1400 | 1400 | 1400 | 1400 | |
| ❑ | 600 | 400 | 200 | 0 | |

✳ Calories required to maintain current weight
✢ Energy (food intake)
❑ Energy deficit

By the time we get to W3, she has lost more weight and now needs only 1600 calories to maintain it, so that the energy deficit is only 200 calories per day. This will produce weight loss of about 200g (just under 1/2lb) per week – so her weight loss slows even more.

At W4, her weight now requires only 1400 calories a day to maintain. Since she is taking in 1400 per day, she is in neutral energy balance and her weight remains constant. To lose any more weight she has three options: to reduce her energy intake even more, say to 1200 calories per day; increase her energy expenditure through exercise, or both.

This pattern explains why weight loss is easy at the beginning, but gets more difficult over time. The key is to be patient and to accept smaller weight losses as you near your goal waist measurement. It's also important to accept that your weight loss may vary quite a lot from week to week. So if you do well one week and have a more modest loss the next, don't worry. As long as the overall trend is down, you are making good progress.

## How do I overcome negative thoughts?

Years of unsuccessful dieting, unkind comments and unhappiness about your body image can easily lead to feelings of despondency and gloom at any mention of weight loss. Then you end up in the awful Catch 22 of eating more because you feel depressed about your weight, and then hating yourself because you are not in control.

It is, therefore, very important to use cognitive therapy to support what you are doing in terms of diet and physical activity. Cognitive therapy is just a fancy way of saying that you should learn how to think positively about things, rather than anticipating failure. If you constantly remind yourself of the health benefits of eating well and getting your weight under control, you are more likely to stay with it. So how do you turn negative feelings into positive ones?

One way is to always counteract any negative thought with a positive one. For example, when you think: 'I'll never do this – it's going to take forever,' turn this into a positive thought such as: 'It's already working and it will go on doing so as long as I'm patient and realistic and don't expect to achieve things overnight' or 'I may have only lost a small amount so far, but I have already reduced my health risks and I feel heaps better'.

Share your aims and aspirations with friends and family – invite them to become involved in helping you. Mark your progress along the road to a healthier weight by rewarding yourself with, say, a new CD, some perfume or some new clothes. Be good to yourself and recognise that life will get better because you are now in control of the problem – not the other way around.

## How do I maintain my weight loss?

Everyone knows that most people who lose weight, even large amounts – eventually put it all back on again. There are complex reasons for this, but part of the explanation must be that they have not really grasped the importance of the energy equation. Many put the weight back because they go back to their old ways of eating and stop being active. They somehow think that the problem is now fixed! *But the problem is never fixed.* If you have a tendency to put on weight, you must accept that this is a lifelong tendency. You can certainly learn how to manage it more effectively, but if you take your eye away from the prize, you will quickly end up where you were before.

Here are some tips for successful weight maintenance:

- Recognise that your tendency to put on weight is for life.
- Weigh yourself regularly – at least once a week – and make corrections to your weight early. It's easier to lose 1Kg (2.2lb) than 9Kg (20lb).
- Use physical activity as a central part of your weight maintenance.
- Use reminders to alert you to the fact that your weight has gone up a little and you need to make some adjustments to your energy intake. For example, if your weight is stable, wear your favourite jewellery or watch. If it's gone up a couple of pounds, wear an old watch you no longer like, so that every time you check the time you will see the watch and remember why you're wearing it.
- Be vigilant – don't ever take your healthier weight for granted.

## What about drugs?

If your weight problem is severe and you have complications, such as diabetes, heart problems or arthritis, your doctor may decide to prescribe anti-obesity drugs. However, some of the drugs used in the past have been found to be unsafe or inappropriate, and have now been withdrawn by the Medicines Control Agency (MCA). The withdrawn drugs belong to the group known as appetite suppressants and include:

• Phentermine (Duromine, Ionamin)
• Dexfenfluramine (Adifax)
• Fenfluramine (Ponderax)

None of these drugs is now licensed in the UK. Another commonly prescribed appetite suppressant called Diethylproprion (Tenuate Dospan) has also been recommended for withdrawal, but this is currently being considered by the European Commission.

Two drugs that are available for the treatment of severe degrees of overweight or obesity are; Orlistat (Xenical) and Sibutramine.

**Orlistat:** Unlike other drugs, this is not an appetite suppressant. It works by reducing the absorption of fat from the gut and this allows up to 30 per cent of the fat eaten in the meal to pass through the gut undigested. Your body cannot, therefore, use this dietary fat as a source of energy and this will help you lose weight. Scientific trials of Orlistat have shown that it may reduce body weight by up to 10–15 per cent. This degree of weight loss may have a major benefit in terms of risk reduction for heart disease and diabetes. The side-effects are usually minor and consist of flatulence, oily or fatty stools and more frequent bowel motions. These unwanted effects are more pronounced if you continue to eat large amounts of dietary fat, so taking Orlistat is a powerful incentive to stick to your reduced fat diet.

Studies suggest that Orlistat is a safe and effective drug which has the advantage that it works locally in the gut, without being absorbed into the body. Orlistat comes in the form of capsules, which must be taken three times each day with the main meals (breakfast, lunch and dinner). It must only be used in support of other lifestyle measures, not as a substitute.

**Sibutramine:** This was originally developed as an anti-depressant, but was found to have powerful weight-reducing properties. It works by suppressing appetite and creating a feeling of fullness, although it may also have some important beneficial effects on thermogenesis (see p.166).

It produces weight loss of a similar degree to Orlistat and appears to be generally safe, although it may cause a slight rise in blood pressure in some patients. Other minor side-effects include dry mouth, headache, insomnia and dizziness, although these tend to become less marked with time. At the time of writing Sibutramine has not been granted a licence for use in the UK, although it has been used successfully in other countries, including the USA and Germany.

*Note:* Drugs should only ever be used to treat individuals with serious weight problems and only then under the care of an appropriately experienced doctor – preferably a specialist with an interest in obesity and metabolic disorders. Furthermore, drug treatment must only be used as adjunctive therapy – in other words as a support to lifestyle changes, not a replacement. Taking appetite suppressants like smarties and expecting this to solve the problem just will not work. If you want success, you have to make substantive, long-term changes in your eating habits and your physical activity patterns. To repeat: there are no quick fixes.

This has been a long section, so to finish let's just bring together the key points in your quest for a healthier weight:

---

### CHECKLIST FOR A HEALTHIER WEIGHT

✓ Measure your waist and if 80cm (32in) or above – take action
✓ Reduce your fat intake and eat a balanced diet, based around vegetables, fruit, grains and pulses
✓ Reduce your alcohol intake
✓ Eat smart and cook smart
✓ Shop smart – choose foods which have no more than 5g of fat per 100g of product
✓ Get active – choose an appropriate activity and try to do this for a minimum of 30 minutes on most days of the week
✓ Aim to lose around 1–2lb per week
✓ Keep a food and activity diary and monitor your weight and waist measurement
✓ Forget crash diets and 'quick fixes'
✓ Only ever use drugs under expert medical supervision
✓ Aim first for a *healthier* weight – not your cosmetic ideal
✓ Be positive – you can do it!

---

# Action File 6
# Sensible drinking

Moderate drinking – the equivalent of one or two glasses of wine a day – may reduce the risk of a heart attack by up to 50 per cent in women aged 50 and over. However, there is no evidence of benefit in younger women, and heavy alcohol consumption at any age is associated with significant health risks, including road traffic accidents, suicide, stroke, liver disease and various forms of cancer. Alcohol intake is measured in standard units and, despite the recent Government guidelines, safe consumption in women is up to 14 units/week, with one or two days' abstinence. If you need to cut down, start a diary and develop some drinking rules to help you take control. Be realistic about your drinking goals and make the adjustments gradually. Good health!

# Background

The pleasurable effects of alcohol have been known for thousands of years and its consumption, and presumably abuse, has featured in the cultures of our ancestors and in our social and religious traditions. For those of us who enjoy a drink – and that's most of us – the challenge is to find a healthy and enjoyable drinking pattern that allows us to enjoy the positive benefits, whilst avoiding the potentially harmful effects. Most of us manage to achieve this reasonably well, but a growing number of us are consuming far too much alcohol and, as a society, we are paying an increasingly heavy price for the privilege. Alcohol is our most popular drug, but it is also a dangerous one.

### What is alcohol and why is it so dangerous?

Alcohol is a drug and, as with any other drug, it has certain side-effects and is potentially addictive. Alcohol can create both a physical and a psychological dependence and has a well recognised (and sometimes dramatic) withdrawal syndrome. In large enough doses, it can cause damage to virtually every organ in the body. In common with other drugs such as barbiturates, regular use of alcohol gives rise to an increased tolerance, so that over time the drinker needs to drink more to obtain the same effect.

## What happens when we drink?

When we drink, alcohol passes virtually unchanged from the mouth into the stomach; about 20 per cent is immediately absorbed into the bloodstream through the stomach wall, the remaining 80 per cent passes into the small gut where it is absorbed into the bloodstream. The alcohol then passes to the liver where it is broken down into waste products. When the liver has removed some of the alcohol, the remainder passes around the body where it can affect virtually every organ with which it comes into contact.

The amount of alcohol in your bloodstream at any one time depends upon a number of factors:

- **The amount of alcohol drunk:** Obviously the more you drink, the higher the blood levels of alcohol.
- **Your weight:** The same amount of alcohol has a greater effect on a light person than a heavy one. This is because the concentration of alcohol in the bloodstream is greater in a smaller person.
- **The sex of the drinker:** A given amount of alcohol has a greater effect on a women than a man because, on average, women weigh less than men. In addition, women – especially younger women – have a lower proportion of their body weight in the form of water: for men this is usually around 55–65 per cent but for women about 45–55 per cent. Alcohol is, therefore, more diluted in men than women, which is why women have a lower tolerance for the same amount of alcohol.
- **Eating food with alcohol:** The presence of food in the stomach tends to slow down the rate of absorption of alcohol into the bloodstream. This is why drinking on an empty stomach is not a good thing.
- **Speed of drinking:** Obviously, the faster you drink the more rapidly the blood level of alcohol will rise.

## How quickly is alcohol removed from the bloodstream?

Blood alcohol concentration is measured in milligrammes of alcohol per 100 millilitres of blood (mg/100ml). One unit of alcohol increases the blood alcohol level within the first hour by about 20mg in a woman and 15mg in a man. In a healthy person, alcohol is removed from the body by the liver at a rate of about 15mg per hour.

This would mean that if you went to bed at midnight with a blood alcohol level of 200mg (after drinking the equivalent of 10 units) and you drove to work at seven o'clock the next morning, you would be likely to have a blood alcohol level well over the legal limit – 80mg/100mls. This is because in that seven-hour period, your body would have removed about 105mg (7 x 15) of alcohol, leaving you with as much as 95mg still in your bloodstream. Moreover, for the first few hours of your working day, you would be more likely to be involved in an accident and your overall judgement would be poorer than normal. It would be well after noon before the residual alcohol was finally removed from your blood-stream.

## What are units of alcohol?

In order to make alcohol consumption more easily quantifiable, the concept of the standard alcohol 'unit' has been introduced. The basic rules are:

One unit of alcohol is equivalent to –

$^1/_2$ pint (250 ml) of average strength beer

*or*

1 glass (125 ml) of wine

*or*

1 standard pub measure (25 ml) of spirits

*or*

1 measure (25 ml) of fortified wine such as sherry or port

So if you drink three glasses of wine and two gin and tonics, you will have consumed a total of five units. If you do this seven nights a week, your weekly consumption will be 35 units.

The problem, of course, is that beers, wines and spirits come in varying strengths so that these definitions of a standard unit of alcohol can be difficult to apply in practice. For example, one glass of low strength (8 per cent) table wine is equivalent to one unit, but the same amount of strong table wine (16 per cent) is two units.

Here is a simple two-step way to find out how many standard units of alcohol are in a given bottle or can of alcoholic drink. First, multiply the percentage of alcohol content by the volume of liquid in the bottle or can, then divide by 100 if the volume is in centilitres (cl) or by 1000 if the volume is in millilitres (ml). Here are some examples:

**A 75 cl bottle of wine with an alcohol content of 14 per cent:**
14 multiplied by 75 (1050) and divided by 100 = 10.5 units.
Given that there are about 6 glasses of wine in this bottle, the average units per glass are 10.5 divided by 6 = 1.75 units.

**A 75 cl bottle of whiskey with an alcohol content of 40 per cent:**
40 multiplied by 75 (3000) divided by 100 = 30 units.
Each bottle contains 75cl, or 750ml (NB. To convert cl to ml just multiply by 10). Given that there are about 25ml in a standard pub measure, each bottle contains 750 divided by 25 = 30 units. So in this case a standard pub measure of 25ml = 1 unit.

**A 440 ml can of cider or lager with an alcohol content of 8 per cent:**
8 multiplied by 440 (3520) divided by 1000 = 3.5 units.

If you have a calculator, this is a quick way of checking the strength of the drinks you normally choose and adjusting your intake accordingly.

## Am I drinking too much?

One of the problems in suggesting safe levels of consumption is that individuals vary enormously in their tolerance to alcohol; what could be dangerous for one person might be remarkably well tolerated by another. Nevertheless, the general rule is that the more you drink, the more likely you are to suffer from alcohol-related problems.

Before 1995, safe drinking in women was up to 14 units/week, but in December that year the Government revised the guidelines upwards to two to three units/day (effectively up to 21 units/week). Alcohol consumption among women has risen since then, but unfortunately the largest increase has been in younger women for whom the benefits are far less clear. So what is the safe upper limit, 14 or 21 units/week?

Our own research helps to clarify this. In Figure 33 you can see that consumption of alcohol up to 14 units/week is accompanied by a significant lowering in the risk of heart disease (about a third). At higher consumption (15–21 units), however, there is not much further reduction in

*Figure 33* Alcohol consumption, risk of heart disease and hypertension in women

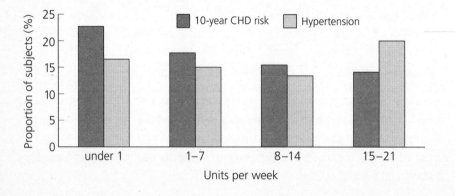

the risk of heart attack, but a 70 per cent rise in the risk of high blood pressure – which is the major risk factor for stroke. In other words, drinking up to 14 units/week provides protection in terms of heart attack risk, but drinking above this level results in a substantial rise in the risk of stroke. Based on these data, I suggest that the 'old' safe-drinking guidelines for women are still the safest i.e:

---

### SAFE DRINKING LIMITS FOR WOMEN

Up to 14 units per week (including two or three days without any alcohol) and a maximum of five units on any one day

---

If you are consistently drinking above this level, you should cut down.

## What are the health benefits of alcohol?

As noted in Chapter 3, evidence would suggest moderate alcohol intake is associated with a 30–50 per cent lower risk of heart disease. Although some wine producers would have us believe otherwise, there is no scientific evidence to support the claim that wine is any better for the heart than other alcoholic drinks. Although alcohol has been shown to reduce the tendency of the blood to clot, the main mechanism by which it is believed to exert its beneficial effect is through an increase in the level of HDL-C discussed earlier.

But, and this is an important caveat, the reduction in heart attack risk associated with moderate alcohol intake is largely confined to women aged 50 years and over. The main reason for this is that an alcohol-associated increase in HDL-C is much more likely to benefit women who are at highest risk of CHD i.e. those over 50 years of age, than younger women. In fact, there is no evidence of benefit in younger age groups; if anything drinking in young women is associated with an *increase* in death rates due to road traffic accidents, violence and suicide.

## Should I start drinking?

Doctors are often asked by non-drinkers whether they should start drinking just to reduce the risk of heart disease. My own view is that they should not; there are lots of other ways to improve and maintain heart health without drinking alcohol and, although it is a drug, it just isn't sensible to use it as a form of medication. Moderate alcohol intake has clear benefits, but there are also important risks associated with alcohol misuse.

## What are the hazards of drinking to excess?

Women develop many alcohol-related medical problems at lower levels of consumption than men, which probably reflects women's smaller body size and lower total body water.

Although the body has a remarkable capacity to recover from the acute effects of alcohol, with high intake over a sufficiently long period, damage to the liver and other organs may become progressive and irreversible. Women are more susceptible to alcohol-related liver damage than men, though precisely why this should be the case is not known for certain. There is also evidence that alcohol increases the risk of breast cancer in women – even at moderate levels of consumption. Other cancers, for example of the mouth, throat, gullet, liver and pancreas are significantly more common in heavy drinkers. Some important areas worth looking at in terms of excess alcohol consumption, are as follows:

### Alcohol and pregnancy

Excessive consumption of alcohol in pregnancy can permanently damage the unborn child. This damage is usually manifest in terms of low birth weight, abnormal growth, mental retardation and a variety of other abnormalities including heart, kidney and skeletal defects. This combination of abnormalities is sometimes referred to as *foetal alcohol syndrome*. Women who drink heavily also have about twice the risk of spontaneous abortion.

Because even very small amounts of alcohol during pregnancy may have a detrimental effect upon the developing child, it is probably sensible for women who plan to become pregnant, or who are already pregnant, to abstain from alcohol or at least to restrict their consumption to an occasional drink, especially in the first three months of pregnancy.

### Alcohol and the heart

On the one hand, regular, moderate alcohol consumption may have some protective effect on the heart, reducing the risk of a heart attack, but only in women over 50. On the other hand, alcohol has a direct toxic effect on the heart, reducing the strength of the heartbeat and sometimes causing disturbances in the normal rhythm of the heart. Women are more at risk than men from alcoholic damage to the heart muscle – a condition known as *cardiomyopathy*, which may result in heart failure (not to be confused with coronary artery disease). Heavy drinking is also an important and common contributor to high blood pressure, although this usually improves if the intake is moderated.

### Alcohol and obesity

A glass of wine contains about 100 calories and a gin and tonic about 140 calories (the same as a large ice-cream). Alcohol is a very efficient producer of calories, but is doesn't supply vitamins or other nutrients; in other words it's just empty calories. This is why heavy drinkers may become very fat and yet be undernourished at the same time. So, if you are trying to lose weight, cutting back on the alcohol is a good way to lose some unwanted calories.

### Alcohol and sex

Evidence shows that heavy drinking reduces the level of sex hormones in the blood, in both men and women. Prolonged heavy drinking may have a direct effect on the ovaries and the testes, but may also damage certain parts of the brain producing a marked reduction in sex drive. Of course, some women and men drink heavily *because* of sexual difficulties, although drinking is only likely to make matters worse. In other words, sexual problems may be both a cause and a result of heavy drinking.

### Alcohol and the brain

You may be surprised to hear that alcohol has a depressant effect on the brain; most people believe it to be a stimulant. The explanation is to be found in the way in which alcohol affects brain function. Alcohol depresses the 'higher centres' – those which control judgement and normal social behaviour – allowing the functions of the lower brain centres (responsible for primitive impulses and emotions), to express themselves. This can produce lack of control, loss of inhibition and aggression, all of which may give the impression that alcohol is having a stimulating effect, when in fact the reverse is the case.

Prolonged heavy drinking may increase anxiety and lead to severe depression. Suicide is about 60 times more common among alcohol abusers than it is generally. Alcohol is not, therefore, a safe or recommended means by which to control either anxiety or depression.

# Action plan

The first thing to do is decide whether you are drinking within the safe guidelines suggested earlier – i.e. up to 14 units per week. If your average consumption is:

**Up to 14 units/week:** You don't need to worry and you probably don't need to read the rest of this section.

**15–24 units/week:** Drinking at this level may not cause any immediate harm, but may increase your chances of having an accident or suffering ill-health in the longer term. Read through hints on how to reduce your alcohol intake, later in this section.

**25–35 units/week:** At this level of consumption there is likely to be physical damage, together with psychological, social, family, occupational, financial or legal problems. You would benefit from reading through the remainder of this section in detail.

**35+ units/week:** Drinking this much is likely to be associated with withdrawal symptoms if alcohol is stopped. Varying degrees of physical damage may be evident. Work through the remainder of this section in detail and, if necessary, talk to your doctor.

It is also useful to ask yourself the following Yes or No questions:

|  | Yes | No |
|---|---|---|
| • Have you ever decided to stop drinking for a week or so, but only lasted a couple of days? | | |
| • Have people annoyed you by criticising your drinking? | | |
| • Have you ever switched from one kind of drink to another in the hope that this would keep you from getting drunk? | | |
| • Have you ever had a drink in the morning during the past year to steady your nerves? | | |
| • Do you envy people who can drink without getting into trouble? | | |
| • Have you had problems connected with drinking during the past year? | | |
| • Has your drinking caused you trouble at home? | | |
| • Have you ever felt bad or guilty about your drinking? | | |
| • Do you tell yourself that you can stop drinking any time you want to even though you keep getting drunk when you don't mean to? | | |
| • Have you missed any days from your work because of your drinking? | | |
| • Do you have loss of memory following a drinking bout? | | |
| • Have you ever felt that your life would be better if you did not drink? | | |
| **Total** _____ | | |

If you have answered Yes to four or more of these 12 questions, the probability is that you already have a significant problem or you are developing one. If you answered Yes to *any* of the questions, this may well indicate that you are beginning to develop alcohol problems, and you should seriously consider ways of cutting down. The following section will help to achieve this.

## Taking control

Let's be clear, the aim of this section is *not* to coerce you into giving up alcohol. It's simply meant to help you to cut down on your drinking and to exert a much greater level of control. You may be under the impression that the only solution to an alcohol problem is to give up drinking completely, but this is not true. There is very good evidence that most problem drinkers can reduce their consumption to amounts which no longer do them harm.

However, if you have already received treatment for alcohol-related problems, or you have already suffered permanent damage from excessive drinking, complete abstinence is probably the only safe course of action for you. Alcohol dependency is a serious and complex problem, and dealing with it is clearly well outside the scope of this book.

There are three major components to the Action plan:

- Monitoring and self-awareness – your drinking diary.
- Your drinking 'rules'.
- Helpful hints to reduce your alcohol intake.

### Monitoring and self-awareness – your drinking diary

Clearly, before you can break a habit completely you have to be aware of it. Much of our drinking (and eating) behaviour is habitual, so having a better understanding of the pattern of your drinking and the circumstances in which you are likely to drink to excess, is a useful first step in taking control. Keeping a weekly drinking diary (see Figure 34) will help you to do this. Start by trying to keep it accurately for the next two or three weeks. You will then be able to construct some drinking 'rules' (see p.185) to help avoid situations where you tend to drink too much.

After this initial period, you need not record the details of your daily drinking, but do record the number of units each day, so that you can calculate your weekly total. You can then monitor your weekly alcohol consumption over the next 12 weeks. This will give you an added incentive to make sure that the target you have set for yourself is achieved during that time.

*Figure 34* Drinking diary

| Day | Time | Hours spent | Place | Who with | Other activities | Money spent | Consequences (if any) | Units |
|---|---|---|---|---|---|---|---|---|
| MON | | | | | | | | |
| | | | | | | | | |
| | | | | | | | | |
| TUES | | | | | | | | |
| | | | | | | | | |
| | | | | | | | | |
| WEDS | | | | | | | | |
| | | | | | | | | |
| | | | | | | | | |
| THURS | | | | | | | | |
| | | | | | | | | |
| | | | | | | | | |
| FRI | | | | | | | | |
| | | | | | | | | |
| | | | | | | | | |
| SAT | | | | | | | | |
| | | | | | | | | |
| | | | | | | | | |
| SUN | | | | | | | | |
| | | | | | | | | |
| | | | | | | | | |
| | | | | | | | Total for week | |

Incidentally, the only thing which determines how intoxicated, ill or addicted you become as a result of drinking, is how much you drink. Myths about mixing drinks or only drinking wine rather than spirits are self-deluding rationalisations. The only thing that matters is the number of units. As far as your liver is concerned, a drink is a drink.

### Your drinking 'rules'

When you have been monitoring your drinking habits for a few weeks, a pattern will begin to emerge which will allow you to draw up your own drinking 'rules'. Simply look at the main circumstances in which you tend to drink to excess, and adopt rules accordingly. An example of some drinking rules for a particular individual are given in Figure 35.

*Figure 35*   Drinking rules

### MY DRINKING RULES

1. I will never drink more than 5 units in one day or a total of 14 units per week
2. I shall not drink at all on Mondays and Thursdays
3. I will stop drinking at lunchtimes
4. I will stop drinking after badminton
5. I will stop drinking with Liz

As you can see, the first rule states that your consumption will not exceed a certain number of units per day or per week. This is important. Whatever your other drinking rules might be, you must have a maximum daily cut-off point (preferably five units) together with a weekly total. Needless to say, these goals must represent a significant reduction in your current drinking habits. Other 'rules' include having one or two days a week when you don't drink at all.

Setting realistic targets is important. The recommended weekly consumption is 14 units and (strictly speaking) this is what you should aim for. However, if you are working through this section in detail, you are probably drinking considerably more than this and so reducing to the recommended levels immediately may be unrealistic. Your drinking rules should, therefore, incorporate slightly different limits which will be easier to achieve, for example three to five units per day or 15–25 units per week (assuming two alcohol-free days). The trick is to reduce your consumption in a stepwise fashion, over a period that you can cope with.

**Helpful hints on reducing your alcohol intake**

Here are some points which will help you to enjoy alcohol, while avoiding the negative effects. Try to use these in combination with your drinking 'rules' and monitor your consumption over the next few weeks.

- Sip your drink slowly and drink smaller measures. Don't try to keep up with other drinkers – your own sensible drinking limits may be substantially lower than theirs.
- Avoid drinking alone.
- Put your glass down between sips – if the drink is in your hand, it's going to end up in your stomach a lot quicker.
- If you drink spirits, dilute them. The longer the drink, the slower the rate at which you will take on the alcohol.
- Use 'spacers' rather than 'chasers'. A spacer is a non-alcoholic drink which you take in between alcoholic ones. This will enable you to space your alcohol consumption over a much longer period of time.
- Try not to use alcohol as a reward. For many people, a stiff gin and tonic at the end of the day is almost a reflex action, but you should try to get out of this habit.
- Working out how much alcohol costs you every month may provide an additional stimulus to cut down – use the money to buy a holiday or a luxury item.
- Pace yourself. Try to decide beforehand how many units of alcohol you intend to consume, and over what period of time you intend to consume them. Try to answer these questions *before* you start drinking.

---

### CHECKLIST FOR CONTROLLING YOUR ALCOHOL INTAKE

- ✓ Record your consumption for a few weeks and set out your own set of drinking rules
- ✓ Rule 1 (the daily/weekly maximum) must be explicit and non-negotiable
- ✓ After a few weeks, you can dispense with the detailed diary, but you should record your daily alcohol consumption in units
- ✓ Be realistic about your drinking goals. If your current alcohol intake is well above the recommended level, reduce your daily and weekly consumption gradually
- ✓ Use the helpful hints above to help control your drinking

Remember: The aim is enjoyable and safe drinking – not abstinence!

# Action File 7
# Coping with stress and insomnia

We all experience various degrees of stress as part of our normal everyday lives. Only when the normal stress response becomes severe or prolonged do the potentially damaging health consequences become apparent. Moreover, there are positive as well as negative forms of stress. Whilst there is no direct evidence that stress leads to heart disease, individuals who already have heart problems may be at risk from sudden stressful life events. Stress-related symptoms include insomnia, irritability, poor concentration, headaches, dizziness and rapid mood change. Lower your stress levels by adopting the lifestyle changes recommended in this section and practising the relaxation techniques. Alternatives such as aromatherapy, yoga and relaxation tapes may also help. Insomnia is another consequence of stress, so practising good sleep hygiene is also important and beneficial.

## Background

Over the last thirty years, it seems that our lives have become faster, tougher and more emotionally and mentally demanding than ever before. The electronic age clearly has its advantages but today many people complain of 'overload' and of having difficulty coping with the extraordinary demands of modern living. Women in particular may have to juggle with a range of competing demands from family, partner, career, domestic and social commitments, etc. And to match our increasingly frantic lives, we have developed a new vocabulary. Expressions such as 'feeling stressed', being 'stressed out' and 'totally stressed' have as firm a place in our everyday language as 'fast foods' and 'software packages'.

## Stress

But what exactly do we mean when we talk about stress? A simple definition is that we feel under stress when we experience the 'stress response'

– a series of physiological and biochemical reactions in the body, which occur as a result of some external stimulus or threat.

## What causes the stress response?

Imagine that you have gone away for a weekend to a remote cottage in Wales and your partner has gone out to pick up some supplies. It has been raining all day and now a strong wind is blowing the rain against the windows. Although it is pitch dark and cold outside, the cottage is warm and you are standing in the kitchen making a cup of tea. As you turn to pick up the kettle you suddenly see a strange and threatening face pressed against the window.

From the moment this happens, striking physical changes are set in motion in your body. Your heart rate and blood pressure increase dramatically and your skin becomes cool and clammy as the blood is diverted away from it to feed the brain and muscles. The palms of your hands become moist and your pupils dilate. A message has been sent from your nervous system to your adrenal glands to secrete the hormones adrenaline and noradrenaline. These hormones increase the force of contraction and the speed of the heart and they also enlarge the airways so that more air can reach the lungs more quickly. Blood sugar (glucose) is released from storage in the liver into your bloodstream in preparation for action (this is an extra supply of fuel that can be burned rapidly). Your blood has also become 'stickier' and more likely to clot should you be injured. In short, you are being prepared to either fight or run – hence the term 'fight or flight' reaction that is often used to describe all these complex bodily changes.

Of course, you don't need to go to a remote cottage in Wales to experience all this. A near miss on the motorway can produce the same, although less severe, pattern of changes. Today, most of the stresses we face are not solved physically by either fighting or fleeing, so the body's stress response has no way to dissipate. We have retained our primitive hormonal and chemical defence mechanisms, but our twentieth-century lifestyle doesn't permit a purely physical reaction to the stress agents we face. In the context of modern life, our ancient 'fight or flight response' is inappropriate – and therein lies the problem.

The stress response is summarised in Figure 36 opposite. Our normal (steady) state is disturbed by what we perceive to be a threat, e.g. the figure at the window, and this produces an initial stress response. If our personality is robust and our coping skills are well developed, we deal

*Figure 36*  The Stress Response*

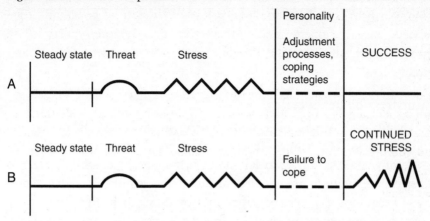

*Source: *Living with Stress* by Cooper – with permission.

with the problem and return once again to our steady state (A). But if we are unable to rationalise the threat and deal with it, we can move into a situation where the stress continues – with all the potentially adverse consequences (B).

## Why is the stress response harmful?

The stress response was originally designed to be a life saving mechanism, to be activated only occasionally. It is, therefore, a perfectly natural phenomenon. However, if the stress response is evoked repeatedly, the body is put into a high state of arousal for long periods, which may be harmful. Exactly how this happens is not fully understood, but it seems the body's defences weaken as a result of prolonged bombardment by adrenaline and other stress-related chemicals. And as stress begins to take its toll, a variety of symptoms – both physical and mental – can result.

In some individuals, the stress response can become addictive. I remember talking to one senior male executive who told me that he deliberately arrived at the airport late, just to feel the buzz of *nearly* missing the plane. Unfortunately our conversation took place in a coronary care unit – it seems his addictive pattern of behaviour had eventually (inevitably, you might say), caught up with him. An extreme example, certainly, but many of us may have less extreme degrees of addictive behaviour. Some of us actively seek out stressful situations, albeit unconsciously, because we miss the state of arousal when we are taken out of it. This is precisely why holidays can be a disaster. When one or other, or both, partners have lived for long periods in a state of constant stress-related arousal, suddenly finding themselves on a remote holiday island away from all the buzz can provoke even greater anxiety, tension and arguments.

## Can stress be beneficial?

Life hands each of us a measure of worry, pressure, success, misfortune and happiness. The way we react to these very different experiences is a result of genetic, cultural, social and environmental factors. Clearly, not all stressful situations are equally harmful; stress is difficult to define precisely because it is perceived differently by different people. What may cause deep anxiety in me, may be an exciting challenge and a necessary motivation for you. Furthermore, it is clear that stress can sometimes be a positive experience. Some of the most rewarding moments in our lives are also stressful; stress can sometimes act as a catalyst to our ambition and add immeasurably to the quality of our lives. It is only when the resulting stress becomes unduly severe or prolonged that problems can arise.

But whatever our individual makeup, there are two things which are certain. Firstly, stress affects *all* of us – it is one of the great hazards of twentyfirst-century living. Secondly, although we can avoid smoking, take regular exercise and avoid fattening or otherwise damaging foods, we cannot avoid stress. We are not in a position to opt out. We are going to experience stress to a greater or lesser extent in normal everyday living. So learning how to deal with stress is becoming increasingly important to our physical and mental wellbeing.

## Stress and illness

There seems little doubt that prolonged stress can lead to physical and mental illness. Scientific evidence shows that our immune system may become weakened, making us more vulnerable to infections such as colds and cold sores. Stress may also contribute to asthma, bowel problems, such as irritable bowel syndrome (IBS), some skin disorders such as eczema and high blood pressure.

## What are the symptoms and signs of stress?

Physical and mental symptoms and signs commonly associated with stress are listed in Table 16 opposite. Do you recognise any of these in yourself, or have others around you mentioned them?

*Table 16*  **Physical and mental symptoms of stress**

| *Physical symptoms* | *Mental (behavioural) symptoms* |
| --- | --- |
| Increased use of alcohol and cigarettes | Rapid mood change |
| Excess sweating | Feelings of anxiety |
| Loss of appetite | Constant irritability |
| Indigestion/heartburn | Feeling unable to cope |
| Constipation/diarrhoea | Loss of interest in life |
| Fatigue | Indecisiveness |
| Recurrent headaches | Loss of a sense of humour |
| Palpitations | Poor concentration and memory |
| Frequent crying | Recurrent fear of disease |
| Feelings of breathlessness at rest | Inability to show feelings |
| Insomnia | Loss of interest in sex |

## Stress and heart disease

Most people believe that stress is a major risk factor for heart disease, but in fact there is little scientific evidence to support this view. One of the difficulties is that, unlike for blood pressure or cholesterol levels, there is no reliable blood test we can do to measure stress levels. But nowadays, the emphasis is not simply on stress in isolation, but on a much broader range of psychosocial risk factors which may increase the risk of CHD and other diseases. These include an individual's mental health (stress, depression and anxiety), personality type, social and economic status, educational attainment and ethnicity (See Table 17 below).

Although there is no shortage of suggestions, very little is actually known about the specific mechanisms by which these factors contribute to heart disease. Furthermore, even if we accept that there is an association between cardiovascular disease and various psychosocial factors,

*Table 17*  **Psychosocial profile of a woman at high risk of CHD**

Lower social class
Little formal education
Higher levels of perceived stress and tension
Prone to hostility and anger
History of depressive illness
Typically a homemaker who feels unsupported socially
If employed outside home, still does all the household tasks
Seldom takes a holiday
If a widow, experiences feelings of loneliness and hopelessness

including stress, we still lack the evidence that this is independent of other well-known factors. For example, people who feel stressed tend to smoke more, take less exercise, drink alcohol to excess and overeat – habits which may in their own right lead to obesity, raised blood pressure and cholesterol levels. Are people with normal risk factor levels still at increased CHD risk if they have high stress levels? Is the response in women the same as that in men? These and many other questions remain unanswered.

## Will reducing stress lower my risk of heart disease?

Athough stress management is an appealing concept and makes sense for a person's overall health and wellbeing, at present we simply don't have the evidence to know whether interventions designed to reduce stress levels will, in themselves, reduce the risk of a heart attack. Studies which have used psychosocial therapies to prevent second heart attacks appear promising, but results are very preliminary and conclusions have to be viewed with caution because of the small numbers of women involved.

What we do know is that if you already have some evidence of heart problems – angina or a heart attack – an acutely stressful event could be dangerous. The likely explanation is that a damaged or diseased heart becomes unstable and the surge of adrenaline produced by a sudden stressful event could be enough to provoke a change in the normal rhythm of the heart.

## How stress-prone are you?

So how well do you think you cope with stressful life events? The Life Events Inventory opposite is based on the life events scale, developed by two American doctors called R.H. Rahe and T.H. Holmes. It uses a list of commonly experienced life events to determine how well you cope and, by implication, your vulnerability to stress. But please understand that this is a *guide* only. It is possible to have symptoms and signs of stress, even though your score may not be especially high.

# LIFE EVENTS INVENTORY*

Place a cross (X) in the 'Yes' column for each event which has taken place in the last two years. Then circle a number on the scale which best describes how upsetting the event was to you, e.g. 8 for moving house.

| Event | Yes | Scale |
|---|---|---|
| Bought house | ____ | 1 2 3 4 5 6 7 8 9 10 |
| Sold house | ____ | 1 2 3 4 5 6 7 8 9 10 |
| Moved house | ____ | 1 2 3 4 5 6 7 8 9 10 |
| Major house renovation | ____ | 1 2 3 4 5 6 7 8 9 10 |
| Separation from loved one | ____ | 1 2 3 4 5 6 7 8 9 10 |
| End of relationship | ____ | 1 2 3 4 5 6 7 8 9 10 |
| Got engaged | ____ | 1 2 3 4 5 6 7 8 9 10 |
| Got married | ____ | 1 2 3 4 5 6 7 8 9 10 |
| Marital problem | ____ | 1 2 3 4 5 6 7 8 9 10 |
| Awaiting divorce | ____ | 1 2 3 4 5 6 7 8 9 10 |
| Divorce | ____ | 1 2 3 4 5 6 7 8 9 10 |
| Child started school/nursery | ____ | 1 2 3 4 5 6 7 8 9 10 |
| Increased nursing responsibilities for elderly or sick person | ____ | 1 2 3 4 5 6 7 8 9 10 |
| Problems with relatives | ____ | 1 2 3 4 5 6 7 8 9 10 |
| Problems with friends/neighbours | ____ | 1 2 3 4 5 6 7 8 9 10 |
| Pet-related problems | ____ | 1 2 3 4 5 6 7 8 9 10 |
| Work-related problems | ____ | 1 2 3 4 5 6 7 8 9 10 |
| Change in nature of work | ____ | 1 2 3 4 5 6 7 8 9 10 |
| Threat of redundancy | ____ | 1 2 3 4 5 6 7 8 9 10 |
| Changed job | ____ | 1 2 3 4 5 6 7 8 9 10 |
| Made redundant | ____ | 1 2 3 4 5 6 7 8 9 10 |
| Unemployed | ____ | 1 2 3 4 5 6 7 8 9 10 |
| Retired | ____ | 1 2 3 4 5 6 7 8 9 10 |

| Event | Yes | Scale |
|---|---|---|
| Increased or new bank loan/ mortgage | _____ | 1 2 3 4 5 6 7 8 9 10 |
| Financial difficulty | _____ | 1 2 3 4 5 6 7 8 9 10 |
| Insurance problem | _____ | 1 2 3 4 5 6 7 8 9 10 |
| Legal problem | _____ | 1 2 3 4 5 6 7 8 9 10 |
| Emotional or physical illness of close family or relative | _____ | 1 2 3 4 5 6 7 8 9 10 |
| Serious illness of close family or relative requiring hospitalisation | _____ | 1 2 3 4 5 6 7 8 9 10 |
| Surgical operation experienced by family member or relative | _____ | 1 2 3 4 5 6 7 8 9 10 |
| Death of husband | _____ | 1 2 3 4 5 6 7 8 9 10 |
| Death of family member or relative | _____ | 1 2 3 4 5 6 7 8 9 10 |
| Death of close friend | _____ | 1 2 3 4 5 6 7 8 9 10 |
| Emotional or physical illness of yourself | _____ | 1 2 3 4 5 6 7 8 9 10 |
| Serious illness requiring your own hospitalisation | _____ | 1 2 3 4 5 6 7 8 9 10 |
| Surgical operation on yourself | _____ | 1 2 3 4 5 6 7 8 9 10 |
| Pregnancy | _____ | 1 2 3 4 5 6 7 8 9 10 |
| Birth of baby | _____ | 1 2 3 4 5 6 7 8 9 10 |
| Birth of grandchild | _____ | 1 2 3 4 5 6 7 8 9 10 |
| Family member left home | _____ | 1 2 3 4 5 6 7 8 9 10 |
| Difficult relationship with children | _____ | 1 2 3 4 5 6 7 8 9 10 |
| Difficult relationship with parents | _____ | 1 2 3 4 5 6 7 8 9 10 |

### Plot total score below:

*Low stress*                                    *High stress*

1                    50                    100

\*Reproduced from *Living with Stress* by Cooper – with permission.

# Action plan

If you're feeling stressed and want to do something about it, here are some general stress management ideas which might help.

## Change your diet

Rushing here and there plays havoc with your diet and digestion. And because you tend to eat on the move, it's often easier to eat 'junk' foods full of fat, sugar and calories. This is why, far from making you lose weight, stress can result in overeating and weight gain. You may also become deficient in essential vitamins and minerals. If you have to eat on the move, read food labels and opt for the low-fat versions (see Part III). It is also a good idea to take a multiple vitamin and mineral supplement.

Another common dietary consequence of prolonged stress is excessive coffee consumption. Heavy caffeine consumption can produce anxiety, restlessness, insomnia, headaches, an increase in pulse rate, high blood pressure and palpitations. It is true that caffeine heightens physical performance, but its effect on mood and intellectual performance is, contrary to popular belief, much less predictable. If you are a heavy coffee or tea drinker, you would be well advised to reduce your consumption or change to decaffeinated.

## Build exercise into your daily routine

It's OK, I've heard all the excuses you can think of – and more besides! I know that getting time to exercise is difficult with the home to run and the children to look after etc. But exercise is a great stress-buster and setting aside time for the gym or the health club will most certainly pay dividends. Apart from being fitter, you will have more energy, sleep better, look better and generally cope better. Collapsing in front of the TV at the end of the day may marginally improve your knowledge of soaps, but it certainly won't lower your stress levels.

## Cut back on the alcohol

One of the early signs of stress is heavy drinking. It may seem as though having a drink helps to calm you down and cope better but, over time, you will develop a tolerance to alcohol which may then turn into a dependence. Drinking may become an escape mechanism, a way of avoiding stressful situations. The need to find temporary respite from stressful life events may also lead to an increased dependence on prescribed drugs like tranquillizers, or a temptation to use non-prescription drugs.

## Make time to relax

We all tend to do it – take on more than we should. But when it comes to the point where you no longer have any time for yourself, it's time to act. We all need some space, even if only for a few minutes each day. So instead of filling every waking moment, learn to say 'No' and mean it. Use the time to develop some new interests and hobbies which take you outside your normal environment.

## Get away

You may not be able to get away for long periods, but sometimes a series of shorter breaks can be just as beneficial. They take less time to plan and you can do them on the spur of the moment. Planning for long holidays can increase your stress levels. You don't have to go to exotic places either; it's the change in surroundings that matters more than the sunshine.

## Keep a sense of perspective

Being under pressure for long periods can easily lead to a loss of perspective. We become so involved in our own world that our horizon narrows and trivial problems seem important. Anyone who has gone through a major life event, such as a heart attack or the sudden death of a partner, emerges with an utterly different perspective on life. Keeping a sense of perspective is an essential part of stress control. As the philosopher Bertrand Russell once said: 'One of the signs of impending madness is the belief that one's work is important. If I were a medical man, I should prescribe a long holiday to anyone who believed that his work was important.'

## Be more self-aware

Learn to recognise signs and symptoms of stress in yourself and don't ignore family and friends if they mention your unusual irritability, mood swings, or drinking; they are usually much better judges of this than you.

## Get plenty of sleep

Insomnia is a very common stress-related symptom. Of course, being anxious and stressed may in itself lead to sleep disturbance, which makes you less able to cope, which then makes you feel more stressed, etc. Breaking the vicious circle can be difficult, but it is essential to set aside adequate sleeping time, even if actually getting the sleep is difficult. Insomnia is discussed in more detail shortly.

## Alternative stress reducers

You may find the following helpful – although, be warned, some are expensive.

*Aromatherapy* is essentially massage accompanied by exotic fragrances and many find this a wonderfully soothing way to release the tension and pressure.

*Health farms* are a good way to get a relaxing weekend away from everything and will usually have facilities for aromatherapy and other stress-reducing aids. The downside is, of course, that they are expensive.

*Herbal remedies,* for example St. John's Wort, are popular as stress reducers, but scientific evidence for their benefit is lacking. More to the point, they may have important interactions with some prescription drugs used to treat heart problems, e.g. Warfarin and Digoxin. For this reason you should on no account take any herbal preparation in combination with prescription drugs, without discussing it with your doctor first.

*Relaxation tapes* are cheaper than the other alternatives given above, although much less fashionable or exotic. Still, it's a much better option than valium or alcohol and you can choose when and where you want to use them. Many people find them very useful but you need to give them a chance and choose carefully.

*Shiatsu massage* is an ancient Japanese adaptation of 'acupuncture through finger pressure' which claims to balance body energies. Whether it does or not, doesn't really matter if you find it helpful. The massage and some of the manipulations can be quite vigorous, so be warned.

*Yoga and Tai Chi* are an excellent way of combining relaxation techniques with muscle stretching and toning exercises.

## Two simple relaxation techniques

In addition to all the above, you may like to try some simple relaxation methods. If you have had heart surgery, or are recovering after a heart attack, you will find these helpful.

### Progressive muscle relaxation (PMR)

PMR is a relaxation technique recommended by the American Heart Association.

Lie down on the floor in a comfortable position with your head and neck supported. Close your eyes and tense each muscle group listed below to about 25 per cent to 50 per cent of maximum tension. Hold the tension for a few seconds as you continue to breathe normally, then slowly release the tension as you focus on the pleasant contrast between tight and relaxed muscles. Contract the muscle groups in the following order:

- Hands and arms
- Face
- Neck and shoulders
- Stomach and abdomen
- Buttocks and thighs
- Calves
- Toes

**Relaxed breathing**

Relaxed, deep, or abdominal breathing is a technique that helps to reduce anxiety and has a calming effect on your emotions. There are four steps:

1. Lie down on your back in a comfortable position and loosen any tight clothing.
2. Inhale through your mouth and exhale through your nose.
3. As you inhale, allow your abdomen to extend. As you exhale, pull your stomach back in.
4. As you inhale, mentally count slowly from one to four. As you exhale, count from one to six or eight.

To begin with, you may find it helpful to place the flat of your hand on the abdomen to actually feel the inhalations and exhalations, until the deep breathing comes naturally. Five or ten minutes is all you need.

# Insomnia

We all have periods when we sleep badly. This may be due to a change in circumstances, such as a new baby, an illness or an operation, or there may be no obvious reason. Usually these periods are short lived and we are able to cope with them. But for some people, occasional sleeping problems can develop into chronic insomnia. About 10 million individuals in this country have significant sleeping problems, although interestingly it is a subject which few people talk about very much. In the USA, up to 50 million people are said to have trouble sleeping. Experts who have studied insomnia attribute the problem to stress, massive information overload and our 24-hour-a-day culture.

## What is insomnia?

There is no standard definition of insomnia, since the amount of sleep required for feeling rested varies enormously between individuals. Some may feel completely rested with as little as four hours sleep while others require a minimum of eight or nine. Essentially, there are two kinds of insomnia:

1. **Sleep onset insomnia** is defined as taking more than 30 minutes to get off to sleep.
2. **Sleep maintenance insomnia** is where you have difficulty staying asleep, as defined by more than 30 minutes' awake-time after falling asleep; or early morning wakening before the desired wake up time, with an inability to get back to sleep.

## The effects of sleep loss

The effects of sleep loss are subject to many popular misconceptions. The belief that everyone has to sleep eight hours a night is a myth. In fact, 20 per cent of the population sleep less than six hours per night. Another significant fact is that our sleep needs decrease with age.

Contrary to popular belief, our ability to tolerate lack of sleep is much greater than we think. Even one night of complete sleep deprivation may have remarkably little effect on how we function at home or at work. In fact, evidence would suggest that most individuals can maintain their usual performance with 60 to 70 per cent of their normal sleep. So if you are an eight-hour-a-night person, you can function quite well on an occasional four or five hours. For moderate sleep loss like this, the perception is as important as the amount lost.

Don't be afraid of insomnia. The less you fear it, the better you will sleep and the better you will feel the next day.

## Why do we sleep?

It is still not known for certain why we sleep, but in the past forty years or so we have learnt a great deal more about the basic physiology involved. Scientists distinguish between two types of sleep: the rapid eye movement (REM) variety – when your eyes are darting about under your eyelids – and the non-REM type, also called orthodox, quiet or slow wave sleep. At night, we alternate between both types of sleep. We dream during REM sleep; non-REM sleep is a deeper type of sleep in which the body repairs itself.

# Action plan

Here are some practical strategies to improve your sleeping pattern. Remember, to get a better night's sleep, you need to prepare during the day and not just before you go to bed.

## Daytime preparation for sleep

- Reduce your consumption of alcohol and caffeine. Contrary to popular belief, alcohol actually disrupts sleep and it should not be consumed within *two hours* of bedtime. Caffeine is a powerful stimulant and this should not be consumed within *six hours* of bedtime (remember that many other foods and drinks contain caffeine besides coffee and tea).
- Drink as little as possible of anything after 8 p.m. to reduce the likelihood of having to get up during the night to pass water.
- Exercise regularly. Regular exercise, including brisk walking, can make a significant contribution to healthy sleeping patterns.
- Give yourself a 'wind-down' period before going to bed. Use this time to think through the day's events and to plan for the morning. Listen to some music, read for a while or watch some TV. A light carbohydrate snack, e.g. some breakfast cereal, may help you sleep.
- Make sure your bedroom is welcoming and conducive to sleep. This is an intensely individual thing. Some people like to have complete silence and darkness, while others might need some background music or noise. Obviously, you need to make sure the bed is comfortable!

## Night-time preparation for sleep

- If you are taking sleeping pills you should aim to reduce and eventually eliminate their use, under your doctor's guidance. Sleeping tablets may help you to get through a particularly difficult period, but they are not a long-term solution. Although you may fall asleep more rapidly than usual, your sleep will be poorer quality. Moreover, when you stop using them you may experience a temporary increase in your insomnia which may be even worse than the initial insomnia. If you have to take a sleeping pill, then you should try to limit this to one per week.
- One of the most common mistakes made by people who suffer from insomnia is to spend too much time in bed. Retire at a regular time each night and reduce your time in bed to no more than six or seven hours – even if it means delaying bedtime by an hour or so.

- Try to get up at about the same time every day (including weekends), even if you have had a poor night's sleep. This helps to maintain a consistent circadian rhythm (the 24-hour internal body rhythm or cycle that keeps humans awake during the day and asleep at night). With time, the hour that you will become drowsy and ready for sleep will become more consistent.

- Don't take naps longer than one hour during the day since this will make you less sleepy at bedtime. However, taking a short nap of *less* than one hour, particularly in the afternoon, might help compensate for a sleep-deprived night and will not usually affect your sleep onset at night.

- Use bedtime for pleasurable relaxing activities and sleep. Don't use your bedroom for any stressful activities such as working or studying. The goal is to associate your bedroom and bed only with relaxation and sleep.

- Go to sleep only when you are drowsy, even if that time comes later than your new delayed bedtime. The important thing is to begin to associate bedtime and your bed with drowsiness.

- When you are drowsy, go to bed and relax for 15 to 20 minutes by reading, listening to music or even watching television until you are *very* drowsy. Then turn out the lights with the intention of *going* to sleep. If you are unable to sleep after 20 minutes or so, *stop trying to sleep!* The harder you try, the more difficult you are going to find it. Instead, open your eyes and read for a while, watch TV, or listen to music until you are drowsy. Then turn out the lights a second time. You can repeat this procedure as often as necessary. You may also find it beneficial to go through the relaxation exercises we discussed in an earlier section. If you are absolutely wide awake, you may find it better to get out of bed and leave the bedroom entirely. Engage in a quiet relaxing activity such as listening to music or reading until you begin to feel drowsy again, and then return to your bedroom with the intention of going to sleep.

Practising proper sleep hygiene is essential if you are going to get over your insomnia problem. If you consistently implement the principles outlined above, the chances are that you will improve your sleeping pattern, even if you still can't manage eight hours a night.

> *Most important of all, don't worry about sleeping – it just makes things worse!*

The key action points for coping with stress and insomnia are summarised below:

---

## COPING WITH STRESS AND INSOMNIA

### Stress

- Learn to recognise signs and symptoms of stress in yourself – don't ignore what others may be telling you
- Pay attention to your diet, reduce alcohol and caffeine consumption and build regular exercise into your daily routine
- Make time to relax and get away from it all – don't be tempted to just soldier on
- Use simple relaxation techniques or try some of the 'alternative' stress reducers such as aromatherapy or massage
- Keep a sense of perspective – it's essential

### Insomnia

- Reduce alcohol and coffee consumption during the day and drink as little as possible after 8 pm
- Don't take naps lasting more than one hour during the day
- Give yourself a 'wind-down' period before retiring and make sure your bedroom is comfortable and conducive to sleep
- Go to bed at a regular time each night and try to get up at the same time every day
- If you can't sleep, get up and do something for a while – listen to music, read, etc. – and then try again
- Don't rely on sleeping pills – they are no substitute for the natural sleeping process
- Don't worry about not sleeping!

# PART III

# Eating for a healthy heart

Eating is one of life's great pleasures. The bewildering variety of new foods now on the market, along with the much wider availability of different ethnic foods, has given us a greater range of choices than ever before. Moreover, being adventurous about eating is not incompatible with eating healthily.

The key to healthy and enjoyable eating is having a basic understanding of nutrition. Being informed about food puts you in control and allows you to make informed choices about what *you* want to eat, as opposed to what the food manufacturers would like you to eat.

The science of nutrition has grown dramatically during the last decade and now provides a firm foundation upon which to make recommendations for healthy eating. The problem is that the amount of nonsense written about diet has increased at the same time. There are few areas of popular writing on health that are so full of fads, false hopes, over-simplification and plain quackery, with the consequence that what most people end up with is a long list of dos and don'ts, with very little understanding of the reasoning behind them. Furthermore, although a number of recent surveys have shown that there is generally a much greater awareness of the importance of healthy eating, they also confirm that equally large numbers of people are still confused about many of the most important nutritional issues. The situation is not helped when even the 'experts' appear to disagree about what we should eat. Scarcely a week goes by without some food scare – such as *e-coli* or BSE – hitting the headlines. Hardly surprising that many people just give up and hope it will all go away.

It is now clear that just as poor nutrition will increase the risk of various diseases, so good nutrition can substantially reduce those risks. My aim in this last part of the book is to give you the essential facts about good nutrition, so that you can get the most enjoyment and the most benefit from your diet. There are three sections:

- Nutrition – the essentials
- Understanding food labels
- Eating for a healthy heart

# Nutrition – the essentials

You may remember from your schooldays that there are five major components of a balanced diet:

- Proteins
- Fats
- Carbohydrates
- Fibre
- Vitamins, minerals and trace elements

## Proteins

Proteins are required for the maintenance and repair of all body tissues.

The major dietary sources of protein are meat, fish, shellfish, eggs, milk, cheese, lentils, peas, beans, nuts, bread and cereal grains. All protein, whether it comes from animal, fish or vegetable sources is made up from the same basic building blocks: *the amino acids*. There are 22 amino acids, and each protein is made up of a different sequence of amino acids, strung together like beads. Different foods contain different types of protein, so it is important to eat a variety of protein sources to ensure that you are getting enough of each amino acid.

It used to be thought that meat, cheese and eggs were essential sources of protein to be eaten in abundance. However, while there is no harm in these foods eaten sparingly, they can contain large amounts of fat; hence the recommendation from a number of expert committees that we should choose fish, pulses and cereals as alternative protein sources.

## Fats

There are several different types of fat, i.e. saturated, monounsaturated and polyunsaturated, but they all contain the same amount of energy (calories), and are all composed of fatty acids. There are about 20 different fatty acids in food, and they all have different properties. It is the relative proportion of the different fatty acids in a fat or oil, which makes it solid or liquid, healthy or unhealthy.

## Fatty acids

Each fatty acid is made up of a chain of carbon atoms, which are joined to each other by a single or a double chemical bond. Fatty acids can be either saturated or unsaturated, depending on their structure. Unsaturated fats are further subdivided into monounsaturated and polyunsaturated fats, depending on whether they have one, or more than one double bond:

- Saturated fatty acids have *no* double bonds in the chain of carbon atoms

$$- C - C - C -$$

- Monounsaturated fatty acids have *one* double bond

$$- C = C - C -$$

- Polyunsaturated fatty acids have *more* than one double bond

$$- C = C = C -$$

The number of bonds in the structure determines the physical properties of the fats. Saturated fats are solid at room temperature, whereas unsaturated fats tend to be liquid. All dietary fats – including oils – contain a mixture of saturated and unsaturated fatty acids. Butter, for example, contains some unsaturated fatty acids, but because about 66 per cent of them are saturated we regard butter as a highly saturated fat. Olive oil, on the other hand, contains about 14 per cent saturates, and 70 per cent monounsaturates (oleic acid) and is regarded as an unsaturated fat.

## Saturated fats

Examples of saturated fats and oils are:

- Dairy fats (butter, cheese, cream)
- Meat fats (beef, mutton, pork, lard, dripping, suet)
- Plant fats (coconut oil, palm oil)
- Processed fats (many fats used in industry to make cakes, biscuits, pies, snacks, sausages and some blended vegetable oils and margarines)

Saturated fats are important because they tend to increase blood cholesterol (and LDL-C) levels and are strongly associated with the development of heart and circulatory diseases. This is why lowering your cholesterol requires a reduction in your intake of saturated fatty acids. In fact, there does not appear to be much of a case on medical grounds for retaining saturated fat in our diet.

## Monounsaturated fats

The main monounsaturated fatty acid in the diet is oleic acid, the main constituent of olive oil. When used in preference to saturated fats, monounsaturated fats – far from increasing the risk of heart attack – can actually protect the heart by reducing the artery-clogging LDL-C. They may also make the blood platelets less sticky and so less likely to form blood clots. This may help explain why many Mediterranean countries, in which large amounts of olive oil are consumed, have relatively low death rates from heart disease. Major sources of monounsaturated fats are olive oil, canola oil, peanut oil, nuts and margarine. Mono-unsaturated oils are liquid at room temperature, but start to solidify at refrigerator temperatures. For example, salad dressings containing olive oil turn cloudy in the refrigerator but are clear when left at room temperature for a while.

### Polyunsaturated fats (PUFAs)

Polyunsaturated fats (PUFAs) tend to have a liquid consistency, whether at room or refrigerator temperature. There are two families of PUFA in the diet: Omega-6 (derived from linoleic acid) and Omega-3 (derived from alpha-linoleic acid).

Omega-6 fatty acids are found in vegetable sources such as sunflower, corn, safflower and soya oils and margarines, grapeseed oil and sesame seeds; Omega-3 fatty acids are found in oily fish, such as mackerel, trout, salmon and pilchards, although they are also present in rapeseed, canola, linseed, soya and walnut oil, pumpkin seeds, meat from grass-fed animals (e.g. beef) and green leafy vegetables. Hence although the Omega-3s are often referred to as 'fish oils', this is a misnomer. The main Omega-3 fatty acids are EPA (eicosapentanoic acid) and DHA (docosahexanoic acid).

Linoleic acid and alpha linoleic acid are both *essential* fatty acids (EFAs) because they cannot be made in the body and must be provided by the diet. Both are needed for growth and the repair of cells and tissues in the body. They are also used to produce a group of substances called 'eicosanoids' which influence a wide range of functions in cells and tissues, including inflammation, blood clotting, immunity and blood pressure. Evidence would suggest that a balance between the two families of PUFA might be more important for health than the actual amounts in the diet. Because we normally get plenty of Omega-6 fatty acids in our diet, we are encouraged to consume more Omega-3s. The easiest way to do this is by eating more fish (see opposite) and choosing rapeseed oil instead of other vegetable oils for cooking.

As we shall see later, a number of expert committees have made specific recommendations about what proportions of fats in our diet should be saturated and what contribution should come from polyunsaturated fats. But remember, all fats contain the same number of calories.

### Fish oils

As we saw earlier, fish oils are a rich source of the Omega-3 polyunsaturated fatty acids, eicosapentanoic acid (EPA), and decosahexanoic acid (DHA), which help maintain a healthy heart. They have been shown to:

- Reduce blood triglyceride levels
- Reduce the risk of blood clots (thromboses) by thinning the blood
- Reduce blood pressure

Studies show that regular consumption of oily fish rich in Omega-3s reduces the risk of a heart attack. Fish consumption may also reduce the risk of sudden cardiac death by protecting against dangerous disturbances in heart rhythm (arrhythmia).

Sources of fish oils high in EPA and DHA include mackerel, trout, tuna, salmon, mullet, sardines, herring, pilchards and anchovies. Not surprisingly, fish oil supplements have become very popular in health-food stores and heavily promoted as a means of preventing heart disease. Some people may well benefit from them, but most of us will do just as well by eating fish rich in Omega-3s as part of our normal diet. Enjoy fish at least twice a week and include one portion of oily fish.

### Trans fats

We saw earlier that saturated fats have no double bonds in the carbon chain, whereas unsaturated fatty acids may have one, or more than one, double bond. Each of the carbon atoms in a fatty acid chain is linked to a hydrogen atom.

In order to convert unsaturated oils into fats that are solid or semi-solid at room temperature, for use in margarine and other spreads, manufacturers use an industrial process called hydrogenation. So when you read that a food product has hydrogenated oil, this simply means that it contains vegetable (unsaturated) fats that have been made saturated. This obviously has implications for heart health, since, as we know, saturated fats tend to increase levels of cholesterol in the blood and, therefore, increase the risk of heart disease. But that's not all ...

Some of the hydrogenated (saturated) fats are of a special type – called trans fats. It turns out that trans fats may have an even more detrimental effect on cholesterol levels than ordinary saturated fats.

Only tiny amounts of trans fats exist naturally in our food supply – just a little in meat and dairy products. So this is a man-made problem arising from commercial hydrogenation. Manufacturers use partially hydrogenated oils in processed foods because they prolong shelf life and improve food texture. Pick up almost any box of snack foods or prepared products from the supermarket shelf and you will see that partially hydrogenated vegetable oil is one of the ingredients. This should alert you to the fact that trans fats are lurking inside.

To limit your intake of trans fats:

- Avoid hard (stick) margarine, fried foods, cakes, pastries, biscuits and savoury snacks that are often high in trans fats.
- Choose soft margarine labelled 'trans free'.
- Avoid food items which have 'partially hydrogenated vegetable oil' as a major ingredient on the label, i.e. near the top of the list.

## Carbohydrates

Carbohydrates are the dietary sources of glucose. They come in two main forms: simple sugars or complex carbohydrates (or starches).

### Simple sugars

Sugars are the simplest form of carbohydrate. They come as one- or two-molecule combinations, i.e:

- One-molecule sugars (monosaccharides) – glucose, fructose and galactose.
- Two-molecule sugars (disaccharides) – sucrose, lactose and maltose.

Of the monosaccharides, glucose (the same substance we call blood sugar), found in nearly all fruits and vegetables, isn't particularly sweet-tasting. Fructose is the sweetest known natural sugar, twice as sweet as sucrose. It is found in honey and some fruits and vegetables. Galactose is rarely seen alone, and exists mainly as a disaccharide combined with lactose.

The disaccharides – which are essentially monosaccharides linked together – always contain at least one molecule of glucose. Sucrose (the familiar white, packet sugar) is made of glucose and fructose. Lactose (milk sugar) is made up of glucose and galactose. Maltose (malt sugar), which occurs when beer is brewed and which is found in malted milk shakes, is made up of two glucose molecules.

The consumption of packet sugar in the UK has fallen substantially in recent years, which suggests that we are all becoming much more aware of the need to reduce our sugar consumption. However, other sources of sugar, such as chocolate and confectionery, continue to make a large contribution to the national diet; in 1998, the average chocolate consumption per head in the UK was 8.5Kg (19lb).

More importantly, an enormous amount of our sugar intake comes from hidden sources. Obviously, food such as cakes, chocolate and pastries have a high sugar content, but so do tinned soups, tinned vegetables, pizzas, frozen prawns, sauces, pickles, tinned meats, cereals and cornflakes. In fact, it is quite difficult nowadays to find any processed food that does not contain at least some sugar.

All types of sugar – caster, granulated, Demerera, icing – provide the same amount of energy (4 calories per gram). Everyone knows that sugar is a direct cause of tooth decay, but when eaten to excess it can also contribute to weight problems. Simple sugars stimulate release of insulin and, since insulin is related to hunger, you will tend to feel hungry again in less time than with complex carbohydrates (see Glycaemic Index p.212). And because in many food sources sugar tends to be combined with fat, this may encourage over-consumption of dietary fat as well as sugar. Although sugar is not the evil substance that some people seem to believe, it is not essential to a balanced diet either. Sweet food occasionally will do you no harm; again it is a question of moderation.

To reduce the amount of sugar in your diet:

- Use less packet sugar in tea, coffee, with breakfast cereals and when cooking. Use an artificial sweetener, reduce the amount, or (better still) cut it out altogether.
- Beware of 'hidden' sugars, in foods like pickles, baked beans, ready-prepared soups, tinned meats, pizzas, some breakfast cereals and so on. Examine the food labels carefully to see how much sugar you are actually taking.
- Many fizzy drinks such as Coca Cola, Pepsi Cola, squashes and some juices contain enormous amounts of sugar. Choose unsweetened varieties.
- Try to cut down on jam, marmalade, honey; all contain large amounts of sugar. Did you know, for example, that jam *must* be 60 per cent sugar in order to be called jam? Choose reduced sugar varieties instead.

### Complex carbohydrates (starches)

Complex carbohydrates (starches), too, are made up of glucose sub-units, but unlike simple sugars do not dissolve in water and need cooking in order to be digested (as, for example, with potatoes and flour). Cooking helps to break starches down into smaller molecules that can then be more easily used as an energy source by your body.

Until recently, complex carbohydrates had become the forgotten nutrient, because for most of this century the British population had been told that starchy carbohydrate foods such as bread and potatoes were inferior to animal products. Bread and potatoes were considered 'energy' foods, in contrast to meat, milk, eggs and cheese, which were regarded as high-protein foods that were essential for normal growth. In the last ten to twenty years, however, our attitude towards the humble starch food has changed dramatically and we now recognise that many foods that are rich in complex carbohydrates play an important part in a healthy diet. Here are some important sources of complex carbohydrates:

- Bread, particularly wholemeal bread.
- Pasta, rice and potatoes.
- Beans, peas and lentils. These are excellent sources of both complex carbohydrates and fibre. Use them in soups, salads, as vegetable dishes or to make meat dishes go further.

### The Glycaemic Index (GI)

Conventional wisdom used to be that all complex carbohydrates were 'good' and all simple sugars were 'bad'. But recent research suggests that this is too simplistic. It is now clear that some carbohydrates are broken down and converted to glucose more quickly than others. The Glycaemic Index (GI) measures how fast the carbohydrate of a particular food is converted to glucose and enters the bloodstream. The index is ranked from 0 to 100: the lower the number, the slower the action.

This is important. Foods that are absorbed quickly – i.e. those with a high GI – produce a rapid increase in blood glucose and insulin levels. Insulin produces hunger, encourages fat storage and is related to the Insulin Resistance Syndrome (p.158). So although foods with a high GI produce a short-term glucose 'fix', in the longer term they may increase your hunger and encourage consumption of higher fat foods. In other words, high GI foods can make you fat.

On the other hand, foods with a low GI result in lower blood insulin levels, are more sustaining and, therefore, help control hunger and appetite. One of the hardest things about going on a diet is feeling hungry much of the time. Choosing carbohydrates with a low GI will satisfy your hunger for longer, making it easier to control your food intake and lose weight.

The development of the GI factor has turned some widely held beliefs upside down. The first surprise was that many starchy foods (such as bread, potatoes, rice and pasta) are digested and absorbed very quickly, not slowly as had always been assumed. Secondly, moderate amounts of many sugary foods are not converted to glucose as quickly as had always been thought. The truth is that many sugary foods have lower GI factors than foods like bread. The GIs for some common foods are shown in Table 18.

*Table 18*   Glycaemic Index – common foods

| LOW<55 | MEDIUM 55–70 | HIGH>70 |
|---|---|---|
| | *Cereals* | |
| Rice Bran, AllBran, Special K, Bran Buds, Oat Bran | Muesli, Kellogg's Just Right, Porridge (oatmeal), Grapenuts, Shredded Wheat, Bran Chex, Kellogg's Mini-Wheats | Cornflakes, Sultana Bran, Rice Krispies, Puffed Wheat, Cheerios, Cocopops, Weetabix |
| | *Breads* | |
| Oat bran bread, pumpernickel, linseed-rye bread, multigrain bread | Pitta bread, hamburger bun, wholemeal bread, light rye bread | Bagels, white bread, French baguette, melba toast, gluten-free bread |
| | *Crackers/Crispbreads/Biscuits/Cakes* | |
| Sponge cake, banana cake, Rich Tea biscuits, oatmeal biscuits | Ryvita, muffins, flan cake, crumpet, angel cake, croissant, digestive biscuits, shortbread, arrowroot biscuits | Donut, waffles, rice cakes, water biscuits, Morning Coffee biscuits, Vanilla Wafers, puffed crispbread |
| | *Grains/Pasta* | |
| Pearl barley, cracked wheat, bulgar, spaghetti, fettucine, vermicelli, noodles, macaroni, linguine, meat ravioli, spirali, tortellini | Gnocchi, brown rice, white rice, couscous, Taco shells, macaroni cheese | Tapioca, Calrose short-grain rice, corn chips, instant rice |
| | *Legumes* | |
| Soya beans, red lentils, lentils (general), kidney beans, butter beans, chick peas, Haricot beans, Pinto beans, baked beans, lima beans, black-eyed beans | Green gram dal, split pea soup, green pea soup | Broad beans |
| | *Vegetables* | |
| Yam, sweet potato, carrots, green peas | Sweet corn, white potato, new potato, beetroot | Pumpkin, mashed potato, French fries, swede, instant potato, baked potato, parsnips |
| | *Fruit* | |
| Cherries, grapefruit, dried apricots, peaches, apples, pears, plums, oranges, kiwi fruit, banana, grapes | Mango, paw paw, raisins, pineapple, fresh apricots, sultanas | Watermelon |
| | *Dairy Foods* | |
| Low fat yogurt, low fat ice-cream, whole milk, skimmed milk, custard | Ice-cream (full fat) | Tofu frozen dessert |
| | *Snack Foods and Confectionary* | |
| Peanuts, jams and marmalades, chocolate | Mars bars, muesli bars, popcorn | Pretzels, dates, corn chips |
| | *Drinks* | |
| Apple juice, grapefruit juice, orange juice | Fanta, cordial | Lucozade, Sports Plus, Gatorade |

Low <55 = Healthy choices   Medium 55–70 = Eat in moderation   High >70 = Are best avoided

As you can see, some foods such as crisps and ice cream have a relatively low GI. But of course they also contain significant amounts of fat – not very healthy and certainly not much use if you are trying to lose weight. So, despite their low GI, they should only be eaten in moderate amounts.

Since lower GI meals are generally preferable, how do you achieve a diet with lower overall GI? Simple:

- Replace very high GI foods with lower GI carbohydrates.
- Include low GI foods at every meal and for snacks.
- Avoid eating high GI foods on their own as snacks.
- Mixing low with higher GI foods will lower your overall GI.

**Dietary fibre**

Fibre or roughage is a special form of carbohydrate. It forms the cell walls of plant foods and is, therefore, the main structural component of all plants, vegetables, fruits and seeds although it varies greatly from one food to another. Dietary fibre is the part of our food that is *not* digested by the body.

Throughout human evolution our daily diet came mainly from plants, unrefined cereals, pulses, root vegetables and fruits, all of which contain large amounts of fibre. For our ancestors, meat and fish were delicacies. Today, not only does a large part of our diet contain no fibre at all, we also eat fewer cereals and much of the bread and cereals we do eat have had most of the fibre refined out of them. Fibre comes in two basic forms: insoluble and soluble.

Insoluble fibre: This is required for a normal, smooth and regular bowel movement. It helps to promote the growth of bacteria, and makes a soft bulky stool. Breakfast cereals, whole grain breads (e.g. wholemeal), nuts, brown rice and bran products, are good sources of insoluble fibre. Vegetables, which contain more moisture than cereals, have a lower total fibre composition, but the proportion of insoluble and soluble fibre is approximately equal. By keeping things moving in the intestine, insoluble fibre may help to prevent a range of bowel disorders, including bowel cancer.

Soluble fibre comes in two main types: *gums*, found particularly in oat products, e.g. oatmeal (porridge), oatbran, beans, lentils and peas, and *pectins*, found in apples, citrus fruits, banana and some vegetables. Soluble fibre dissolves in water and forms a gel in the gut, and may help lower levels of blood cholesterol, especially the harmful LDL-C form. (This cholesterol-lowering effect is, however, relatively modest.)

To increase your daily intake of fibre:

- Eat more bread, especially wholemeal bread which contains twice as much fibre as white.
- Eat more cereals, wholewheat pasta, brown rice, oats including porridge and rye bread.
- Eat more vegetables, especially peas, beans, lentils but also leaf and root vegetables.
- Eat more fresh fruit, which is an important source of dietary fibre, particularly 'soluble fibre'.

It is important to eat a mixture of these different foods to make sure you get a balanced intake of the various types of fibre. *Note*: Increase your fibre consumption gradually; this will help you to avoid bloating and discomfort which may otherwise occur.

## Vitamins, minerals and trace elements

These are sometimes known collectively as 'micronutrients'. There are more than 30 micronutrients essential for health, some of which are shown in Table 19.

Vitamins, minerals and trace elements are essential in your diet so that your body can use the rest of your food effectively. They assist with the absorption and the breakdown of various dietary components, and also the repair and rebuilding of body tissues.

*Table 19*  Micronutrients

| Vitamins | Minerals |
|---|---|
| *Fat-soluble* | Calcium |
| Retinol and carotenoids (Vitamin A) | Chlorine |
| Calciferols (Vitamin D) | Magnesium |
| Tocopherols (Vitamin E) | Phosphorus |
| Phylloquinones (Vitamin K) | Potassium |
| | Sodium |
| *Water-soluble* | Sulphur |
| Thiamin (Vitamin B1) | |
| Riboflavin (Vitamin B2) | *Trace elements* |
| Nicotinic acid | Chromium |
| Pyridoxine (Vitamin B6) | Copper |
| Cobalamins (Vitamin B12) | Fluorine |
| Folic acid | Iodine |
| Biotin | Iron |
| Pantothenic acid | Manganese |
| Ascorbic acid (Vitamin C) | Molybdenum |
| | Selenium |
| | Zinc |

Vitamins are divided into two types; the fat-soluble vitamins found mainly in fatty foods, and the water-soluble vitamins that occur in both fatty and non-fatty foods.

Fat-soluble vitamins (A, D, E and K) are found in meat, fish, dairy products and vegetable oils, although green and yellow vegetables are also sources of vitamins A and K. These vitamins travel in fat, which makes them less fragile than their water-soluble counterparts, so they are better able to survive the cooking pot and processing plant.

Water-soluble vitamins include vitamin C, plus eight B vitamins including folic acid. They are much less hardy than their fat-soluble relatives. Because they are vulnerable to heat, they are often broken down in cooking and processing, and some can also be destroyed by light. Fortunately, they are relatively easy to replace. With few exceptions (like vitamin B12), the water-soluble vitamins are present in a wide variety of foods, either naturally or as synthetic fortifiers.

Minerals and trace elements have a vast array of complex biochemical interactions, both with themselves, normal dietary constituents and the various vitamins. This is a fascinating subject in its own right and for those who would like to read more, there are plenty of books available.

From a practical point of view, you need only know that a well-balanced diet should provide you with all the micronutrients you need. Choosing a variety of foods from each of the five food groups (see Balance of Good Health p.222) will help ensure you meet your needs. If you feel that some elements of your diet are not well covered, or that your eating patterns or lifestyle do not allow you to achieve the balanced diet you would like, you may wish to consider taking a general vitamin supplement. There are many of these available, and you should choose a one-a-day multivitamin and mineral combination in amounts close to the Recommended Daily Allowances (RDA), rather than individual high-dose supplements. Specific vitamin supplements for heart disease are discussed below.

### Vitamins and heart disease

As we saw in Chapter 3, there is some evidence that certain vitamins may have a specific protective effect in relation to heart disease. The main candidates are antioxidants (vitamins E, C and beta-carotene) and folic acid.

*Antioxidants.* All cells in the body use oxygen to burn the carbohydrates, fats and proteins that give them energy. Just as a car creates exhaust fumes from burning petrol, the cells in the body produce by-products called free radicals. These are highly reactive molecules that can range throughout the body causing damage to cells and to DNA – the cell's genetic material – and have been linked to ageing and an increased risk of heart disease and cancer. To combat these effects, the cells utilise a range of antioxidants (chemicals which limit the damaging effects of free radicals). Some scientists believe that, as people age, the body becomes less efficient at producing antioxidants, thus making them more prone to various diseases.

The main antioxidants are beta-carotene (a form of vitamin A), vitamin C and vitamin E. They may help prevent heart disease by reducing the oxidation of LDL-C – the 'bad' cholesterol – thereby limiting the build-up of fatty plaque in the arterial wall. The RDAs for these antioxidants, their main dietary sources and the evidence for protection against heart disease, are shown in Table 20 below.

So should you take specific antioxidant vitamin supplements to help your heart? As you can see from the table, all these antioxidants are readily available from a normal balanced diet and the only one for which there may be a case for supplementation is vitamin E. The problem is that the ideal dose required for prevention – both in those with and without heart disease – has yet to be defined. Until we have more information, my

*Table 20*  **Antioxidants and heart disease**

| Nutrient | Recommended Daily Intake (RDI) | Dietary sources | Evidence |
| --- | --- | --- | --- |
| **Vitamin E** | 30 IU | Vegetable oils (soya, corn, olive, cottonseed, safflower, and sunflower), nuts, sunflower seeds, wheat germ | Doses of 100-800 IU may lower heart disease risk by 30%–40% |
| **Vitamin C** | 60 mg | Citrus fruits, strawberries, tomatoes, cantaloupe, broccoli, asparagus, peppers, spinach, potatoes | Consuming more than the RDI in supplement form has not been found to prevent heart disease |
| **Beta-carotene** | None available | Dark green, yellow, and orange vegetables including spinach, collard greens, broccoli, carrots, peppers, and sweet potatoes; yellow fruits such as apricots and peaches | No association between beta-carotene *supplements* and heart disease risk, but some evidence that carotenoid-rich *foods* protect against heart disease |

own view is that a modest dose of vitamin E as a supplement is unlikely to do any harm – and may well do some good. Ask your pharmacist for details.

*Folic Acid.* Homocysteine is a normal breakdown product of dietary protein and, as discussed in Chapter 3, elevated blood levels of homocysteine may increase the risk of heart attack. Blood homocysteine levels are strongly influenced by diet, as well as genetic factors. Conversely, there is some evidence that B vitamins may lower elevated homocysteine levels and so reduce the risk of heart disease. The dietary components with the greatest effects are folic acid and vitamins B6 and B12. The problem is that, as yet, no properly controlled study has shown that taking folic acid or other vitamin B supplements, will reduce the risk of heart disease, or that taking these vitamins has any effect on further heart problems in those who already have the disease. Moreover, folic acid and B vitamins are readily available from a balanced diet. Good sources of folate and B vitamins include leafy green vegetables (e.g. spinach, broccoli), whole-grain breads and cereals, rice, nuts, milk, eggs, cheese, meat and fish, poultry, liver, berries, potatoes, citrus fruits and juices. Some foods, for example cereals and bread, have added folic acid – look for the Folic Acid Mark.

If you are eating a balanced diet, rich in these food sources, there is probably little advantage to be gained from taking B-vitamin supplements. However, if you have reason to think your diet isn't adequate, taking additional folic acid and B vitamins is well worth considering. Ask your pharmacist for advice.

# Understanding food labels

Most of the products in your local supermarket or shop have some nutritional information printed on the label or the packet, although the amount of detail is variable. Before placing an item in your basket, it is a good habit to scan the label. Food manufacturers are very smart and they know exactly how to use words, colours and pictures to entice you into buying their brand or product. But by applying some basic nutritional knowledge, you should have no problem in sifting the fact from the fiction and making smart food choices.

When checking food labels, think about how the product might fit into your overall diet and see how a food's nutrient content contributes to the nutrients you are most interested in. For example, if you are interested in lowering your blood pressure, you will be particularly interested in the sodium content of the food.

*Table 21*   Daily guideline intakes for women

| | |
|---|---|
| Calories | 2000 |
| Fat | 70 g |
| Saturated fat | 20 g |
| Sugar | 50 g |
| Sodium (salt) | 2.0 g |
| Fibre | 16 g |

It is also worth bearing in mind the Daily Guideline Intakes for the major dietary components (see Table 21). Of course, these are *average* guidelines only. A very active woman will need more and someone who is working towards losing weight will need less. The amount we eat may also differ from day to day, in accordance with our activity levels.

## What each nutrient means

Here is a typical food label taken, in this case, from a tin of baked beans (see Figure 37). Note that manufacturers list the values for each ingredient according to the amount per average serving, or per 100 g of product. The latter is generally more useful, because it allows you to make easy comparisons with other food products.

*Figure 37*   **A typical food label**

| NUTRITION INFORMATION | | |
|---|---|---|
| Typical Values | Amount per 100g | Amount per Serving (207g) |
| Energy | 312kJ/75kcal | 646kJ/155kcal |
| Protein | 4.7g | 9.7g |
| Carbohydrate (of which sugars) | 13.6g (6.0g) | 28.2g (12.4g) |
| Fat (of which sugars) | 0.2g (Trace) | 0.4g (0.1g) |
| Fibre | 3.7g | 7.7g |
| Sodium | 0.5g | 1.0g |
| Per serving (207g): 155 Calories 0.4g fat | | |

*Energy (Kcals or KJ):* The amount of energy measured as calories (or joules) that you will get from the food.

*Protein (g):* Important for tissue growth and repair. We usually get more than enough, so you don't need to worry too much about this.

*Carbohydrate (g):* This is mainly starches (complex carbohydrates) and sugars. Some labels will tell you how much there is of each, some will just give the total carbohydrate. Try to choose foods with carbohydrates that are mainly in the form of starches, which tend to have a lower glycaemic index, (most breads, cereals, pasta, oats etc) rather than simple sugars. In the example given, around half the total carbohydrates are simple sugars.

*Sugar (g):* Even if you don't add sugar to foods, there's still a lot to be found in processed foods. In lists of ingredients, words like honey, glucose, dextrose and corn syrup are all different types of added sugar. The nutrition panel may list the carbohydrate content followed by 'of which sugars' or 'added sugars'. This refers to all the sugars in the product, whether natural or added. As a rule of thumb, if the sugar content is 10g per 100g of product, this is 'high' and around 2g is 'low'. You can see in the example label above, that this product has 13.6g of carbohydrate, of which 6.0g are sugar. The manufacturers also make a 'Weight Watchers' version which contains much less sugar.

*Fat (g):* The total amount of fat in the food. This is sometimes broken down into saturates, monounsaturates and polyunsaturates. Try to choose foods that are lower in total fat and saturates. When choosing oils, for example cooking oils, go for ones that are also rich in monounsaturates. As a rule of thumb, choose foods which have no more than **5g of fat per 100g of product.** These baked beans are very low in total fat (0.2g) of which only a trace is saturated.

*Sodium (g):* Most of the sodium in food comes from salt (sodium chloride). As a large amount of the salt we eat comes from processed foods, checking labels for sodium content is important. Although the amounts of sodium seem quite small compared with other food groups, small amounts matter – particularly if you are trying to lower your blood pressure. In general, 0.5g of sodium per 100g of product is a lot, and 0.1g a little. In addition:

- Sodium (salt) free: contains less than 0.005g (5mg) per 100g
- Very low sodium: contains less than 0.035g (35mg) per 100g
- Low-sodium: contains less than 0.14g (140mg) per 100g

In the example label given, the sodium content is quite high, so you would need to bear this in mind if you were trying to cut down on your salt intake.

*Fibre (g):* The total amount of fibre in food (both soluble and insoluble). The rule of thumb for fibre is that 3g per 100g of product is 'high' and 0.5g is 'low'. In the example given, the fibre content is good at 3.7g per 100g.

So you can see that baked beans are a highly nutritious food item, containing only a trace of saturated fat, a good helping of dietary fibre and a moderate amount of carbohydrate for energy. The reduced sugar and sodium versions of this product would be of interest to those who are losing weight or watching their sodium intake.

# Eating for a healthy heart

A healthy, balanced diet plays an essential part in the prevention of heart disease, obesity and a variety of other diseases, including diabetes, cancer and osteoporosis. Because different foods contain many different types of nutrients in different proportions, no single food can provide you with all the nutrients you need for a balanced diet. This is why variety in your diet is so important: it allows you to obtain different nutrients from a wide variety of sources, so that a correct balance is achieved. You can best achieve this by choosing foods from each of the five main food groups every day, i.e:

> *Group 1*: Bread, cereals, pasta, potatoes, rice etc
> *Group 2*: Fruit and vegetables
> *Group 3*: Milk and dairy products
> *Group 4*: Meat, and fish
> *Group 5*: Foods containing fat and sugar

Table 22 (p.222) provides a framework which can form the basis of a healthy diet for the whole family.

## The Mediterranean diet

Mediterranean countries such as Greece and Southern Italy, have much lower death rates from heart disease than the populations of Northern European countries. As a result, the Mediterranean diet has attracted a great deal of interest as a healthy eating plan for reducing the risks of heart disease. Countries that border the Mediterranean Sea are culturally diverse and, although their traditional diets vary somewhat from one country to another, there are some common elements. Figure 38 (see p.223) shows the basic components of the diet and the frequency with which they tend to be consumed.

*Table 22*  The balance of good health

Different amounts will suit different people – according to age, activity, sex etc. Not designed for the under-fives.

| Food group | Main nutrients | What to choose | How much | Other points |
| --- | --- | --- | --- | --- |
| Bread, potatoes & other cereals | Carbohydrate (mainly starchy), fibre, B vitamins, potassium, selenium, some protein, iron calcium, vitamin E, antioxidants | All kinds of bread, pasta, rice, noodles, breakfast cereals, potatoes, yams, oats and grains. Include 3 or more daily servings of wholegrain types | Make these the basis of each meal, but limit added fat. A serving is: slice of bread; $1/2$ bagel; bowl of cereal; 42g ($1^1/2$oz) cooked rice, 56g (2oz) pasta or noodles. Have at least 6 servings each day | Most people would benefit from eating more of these foods. They are filling, nutritious and not as 'fattening' as is commonly believed Tea cakes, oatmeal biscuits, cereal, crackers, and malt loaf make good snacks |
| Fruit & vegetables | Vitamin C, folic acid, beta-carotene, fibre, magnesium, potassium,some carbohydrate, iron, calcium, antioxidants | All types – fresh, frozen, canned, dried, juices. Choose a variety of different types and colours each day | Aim for at least 5 portions every day. A portion is: 2 tbsp vegetables, 2–3 tbsp cooked fruit, side salad, medium fruit, glass of juice, 1tbsp dried fruit | Most people could benefit from eating more. Diets rich in fruit and vegetables can help protect against chronic disease and aid weight control |
| Milk & dairy foods & alternatives | Calcium, protein, vitamin B2, B12, zinc, vitamins A & D | Opt for lower fat varieties e.g. reduced fat milks, yogurt, fromage frais & cheeses. Calcium fortified soya milk or yogurt | Eat or drink a moderate amount, 2–3 servings daily. A serving is 220ml (8fl oz) milk/soya milk, small pot yogurt, 28g (1oz) cheese, 112g (4oz) cottage cheese | A good calcium intake throughout life (especially during adolescence and early 20s) helps reduce risk of osteoporosis |
| Meat, fish & alternatives | Protein, iron, B vitamins, zinc, magnesium, potassium | Lean and trimmed meats, poultry, all types of fish, eggs, beans, split peas and lentils, nuts, meat substitutes, e.g. tofu, TVP | Eat moderate amounts e.g. 2 servings a day. A serving is: 56–84g (2–3oz) meat, 112g (4oz) fish, 1–2 eggs, 3 tbsp cooked beans/lentils | Important to help prevent iron deficiency: common amongst women of child bearing age |
| Foods rich in fat and/ or sugar | Fat, including some essential fats, vitamins, minerals & sugars | Unsaturated oils, e.g. olive, rape-seed, sunflower, soya and their spreads. Use fats sparingly when preparing food | Eat foods high in fat and/or sugar in small amounts; especially those high in saturated fat. Look out for lower fat alternatives to spreads, dressings & ready meals | Keep any sugary foods and drinks to mealtimes to reduce risk of tooth decay. Diets high in saturated fat are linked to increased risk of heart disease |

*Figure 38*  The Mediterranean food pyramid

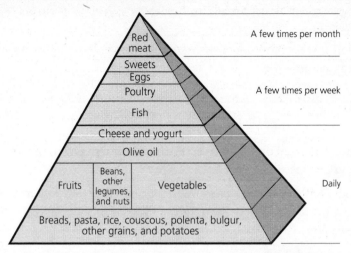

The diet is based around a generous intake of fruits, vegetables, grains, legumes and nuts, which make up around one half of the diet. The principal fat is olive oil, and most people eat some yogurt and cheese each day as well. Fish, eggs, poultry and sweets are consumed sparingly and red meat just a few times a month. What makes this a heart-healthy diet?

1. Olive oil is rich in the monounsaturated fat oleic acid. Mono-unsaturated fats tend to increase HDL-C, whilst reducing the harmful LDL-C and triglycerides. The net result is a reduced risk of heart disease.
2. Fruits, vegetables (particularly the green leafy variety), whole grains, olive oil and nuts are rich sources of antioxidants and B vitamins, including folic acid.

Overall, the traditional Mediterranean diet encourages consumption of plant proteins, rather than animal proteins, whereas the typical Western diet tends to do the reverse. If you look at this food pyramid carefully, you can see that it closely resembles the British Diatetic Association recommendations for healthy eating in Table 22. Of course, Mediterranean people also enjoy the occasional glass of red wine, which may contribute further to their low rates of heart disease!

The Mediterranean diet is a healthy approach to eating if your weight is normal. However, if you are trying to lose weight, the heavy consumption of olive oil may contribute a lot of unwanted calories and cause your weight to increase. And bear in mind that because the weather is generally good, people living in the Mediterranean spend more time working out of doors, walk rather than drive, and spend less time slouched in front of the TV.

To finish this section, let's now summarise the key points in eating for a healthy heart:

---

### THE HEALTHY HEART DIET

- Eat a balanced diet with recommended amounts from the five main food groups

- Reduce your total fat consumption, and saturated fats in particular. Choose foods less than 5g fat/100g of product and beware of *trans* fats

- Avoid foods high in cholesterol (e.g. shrimps, liver and eggs) if your own cholesterol level is raised. Although dietary cholesterol makes only a very small contribution to blood levels, it is best avoided if you are trying to lower it

- Increase your consumption of fish. Marine oils are rich in Omega-3 fatty acids and these will help to reduce total and LDL-cholesterol, as well as reducing the blood clotting tendency

- Choose complex carbohydrates (starches) rather than sugars and avoid those with a high Glycaemic Index

- Reduce your salt consumption. Salt is linked to the development of high blood pressure, which is in itself a major risk factor for heart disease and stroke.

- Eat plenty of foods rich in B vitamins, folic acid and antioxidants, i.e. leafy green vegetables (e.g. spinach, broccoli), whole grain breads and cereals, rice, nuts, milk, eggs, cheese, meat and fish, poultry, liver, berries, potatoes, citrus fruits and juices, brightly coloured vegetables and fresh fruits

- Take a regular general mineral supplement, and consider additional supplements such as Vitamin E, folic acid and B vitamins if necessary

- Increase your consumption of fibre, particularly soluble fibre

- If you drink, consume regular, moderate amounts of alcohol

# And finally...

My aim in this book has been to provide a concise summary of subjects related to heart disease in women, ranging from drugs and surgery, through the menopause and HRT, to the benefits of antioxidants and the Mediterranean diet. Because it spans such a broad canvas, I am aware that there are areas which could have been covered in more detail and others which I have omitted altogether. But one cannot say everything. I hope that all readers will find something of interest and – hopefully – a lot more. To conclude, here are a few parting thoughts.

Firstly, there are two ways of reading this book; as a glass which is half-empty, or half-full. If you see it as half-empty, then the contents will seem like a long list of dos and don'ts which will inhibit your lifestyle and demand long-term self-denial. But if you read it as a glass half-full, you will see it not only as a means of reducing your long-term health risks, but also as a way to get more out of life, to be fitter and physically active well into old age.

Secondly, whether you already have heart disease or not, you really can change your life by making *modest* changes in your diet and physical activity. You don't need to become a marathon runner to get the benefits of physical activity and you don't need to exist on a diet of cucumber sandwiches and mineral water to benefit from sensible eating. Far better to make modest changes which are sustainable, than to make big gestures which will invariably last about six weeks.

Finally – and most important of all – remember that heart disease is not inevitable. You are not the passive recipient of some malign fate that selects certain women to develop the disease and others not. It's a disease like any other disease; the problem should not be accepted, it should be attacked. By applying the principles set out in this book and making informed choices, you *can* do something positive to prevent it. I wish you good heart health!

# Appendix 1
# Useful addresses

## General information about heart disease

Several organisations in the UK can provide further information and advice about all aspects of heart disease and its treatment.

British Heart Foundation (for England and Wales)
4 Fitzhardinge Street
London W1H 4DH
Tel: 0207 935 0185
Website: www.bhf.org.uk

British Heart Foundation (for Scotland and Northern Ireland)
45a Moray Place
Edinburgh EH3 6BQ
Tel: 0207 935 0185
Website: www.bhf.org.uk

The Family Heart Association
7 North Road
Maidenhead
Berkshire SL6 1PE
FHA: Helpline 01628 628 638 (Tuesday-Friday 9a.m.-3p.m.)
E-mail: ad@familyheart.org
Website: www.familyheart.org

The equivalent organisation in the US is:

US National Heart, Lung and Blood Institute
Educational Programs Information Center
PO Box 3015
Bethesda, Maryland 20824-0105
Website: www.americanheart.org

## Cardiac rehabilitation

For information about rehabilitation programmes throughout the UK, contact:

> Cardiac Rehabilitation Group
> Genesis 6
> University of York
> York YO10 5DG
> Tel: 01904 434127
> Fax: 01904 434102
> E-mail: jw1@york.ac.uk
> Website: www.cardiacrehabilitation.org.uk

## Alcohol

> Drinkline: National Alcohol Helpline
> Helpline 0800 917 8282 (weekdays 9am–11pm; weekends 6p.m.–11p.m.)

Drinkline is for anyone who needs information or help about alcohol. It will provide information and help to callers worried about their own drinking, support the family and friends of people who are drinking and advise callers on where to go for help.

> Al-Anon Family Group UK and Eire
> 61 Great Dover Street
> London SE1 4YF
> Tel: 0207 403 0888 (confidential helpline)
> E-mail: alanonuk@aol.com
> Website: www.hexnet.co.uk/alanon

Al-Anon is a Fellowship for relatives and friends of problem drinkers. Members meet in confidence, share experiences and learn how to cope with the problems which arise whether the drinker is still drinking or in recovery. Al-Ateen is a part of Al-Anon that is especially for teenagers who have a parent or other close relative with a drink problem.

Alcoholics Anonymous (AA)
P.O. Box 1
Stonebow House
Stonebow
York YO1 7NJ
Tel: 01904 644026
Fax: 01904 629091
Website: www.alcoholics-anonymous.org.uk/

Alcoholics Anonymous is an informal society of more than 2 million recovered alcoholics in the UK, Canada, the United States and other countries. These men and women meet together in local groups, which range in size from a handful in some localities, to many hundreds in larger communities. They provide support and hope for each other through shared experiences and help others recover from alcohol addiction. There are many local groups throughout the country and the central office or the website can provide details of a group near you.

## Diabetes

Diabetes UK, is the charity for people with diabetes. It provides support and information for diabetics, including up-to-date information about treatment and research. Contact them at:

Diabetes UK Central Office
10 Queen Anne Street
London W1G 9LH
Tel: 020 7323 1531
Fax: 020 7637 3644
E-mail: info@diabetes.org.uk
Website: www.diabetes.org.uk

# DVLA

To inform the Driver and Vehicle Licensing Agency (DVLA) about a heart condition or operation, contact:

> Drivers Medical Unit
> DVLA
> Swansea SA99 ITU
> Tel: 0870 600 0301 (Monday–Friday 08:15a.m.–16:30p.m.)
> Website: www.dvla.gov.uk

# Exercise

*Heart rate monitors*
If you are interested in purchasing a heart rate monitor, you can visit your local sports shop or contact:

> Leisure Systems International Limited
> Northfield Road
> Southam
> Warwickshire CV33 OFG
> Tel: 01926 811611
> Fax: 01926 816105
> E-mail: Isisales@Isi.co.uk
> Website: www.polar.fi

# Hypertension

> British Hypertension Society
> Information Service
> Blood Pressure Unit
> Department of Medicine
> St George's Medical School
> London SW17 ORE
> Tel: 020 8725 3412
> E-mail: bhsis@sghms.ac.uk
> Website: www.hyp.ac.uk/bhsinfo

Recommended devices for home blood pressure measurement available from:

Omron Healthcare Ltd
18-20 The Business Park
Henfield
West Sussex BN5 9SL
Tel: 01273 495033
Fax: 01273 495123
E-mail: amy@hhl.co.uk

## Menopause

Several organisations in the UK provide information and support in relation to gynaecological problems and the menopause.

Amarant Trust
1st Floor Sycamore House
5 Sycamore Street
London EC1Y OSG
Tel: 0207 401 3855
Helpline: 01293 413000
E-mail: amarant@marketforce-communications.co.uk

Women's Health Concern
Wellwood
North Farm Road
Tunbridge Wells
Kent TN2 3DR
Tel: 0208 780 3916
Helpline: 0208 780 3007

## Nutrition

For useful information on all aspects of diet and nutrition contact:

British Nutrition Foundation
High Holborn House
52–54 High Holborn
London WC1V 6RQ
Tel: 020 7404 6504
Fax: 020 7404 6747
E-mail: postbox@nutrition.org.uk
Website: www.nutrition.org.uk

## Osteoporosis

For further information about osteoporosis contact:

> The National Osteoporosis Society (NOS)
> PO Box 10
> Barton Meade House
> Radstock
> Bath BA3 3YB
> Tel: 01761 471771 (general enquiries)
> Helpline: 01761 472721 (for medical enquiries)
> Fax: 01761 471104
> E-mail: info@nos.org.uk
> Website: www.nos.org.uk

## Polycystic Ovarian Syndrome (PCOS)

Women with polycystic ovaries (PCOS) have established their own self-help group called *Verity*. They provide information and support for women with PCOS, togther with up-to-date information on the latest research into the condition. Contact them at:

> Verity
> The PCOS Self-Help Group
> 52-54 Featherstone Street
> London EC1Y 8RT
> Tel: 020 7251 9009
> E-mail: pcos-uk-subscribe@eGroups.com (to share experiences with other women), or membership@verity-pcos.org.uk for information about membership.
> Website: www.verity-pcos.org.uk or www.pcosupport.org

## Smoking cessation

> QUITLINE®
> This is a telephone helpline for people who want to stop smoking. There is special support available for pregnant women, and five Asian language lines.
>
> Ring QUITLINE – FREEPHONE 0800 00 22 00

ASH (Action on Smoking and Health)
16 Fitzhardinge Street
London W1H 4DH
Tel: 0207 739 5902
Website: www.ash.org.uk

## Stroke

The Stroke Association has developed a wide range of Information
and Education Service locations throughout the UK. Trained staff and
volunteers will answer your questions or put you in touch with appropriate people and organisations. They can be contacted at:

Stroke Advisory Service
Stroke House
123 Whitecross Street
London EC1Y 8JJ
Tel: 020 7566 0300
E-mail: advisory@stroke.org.uk
Website: www.stroke.org.uk

# Appendix 2

# Your cholesterol-lowering diet

**In general, try to choose foods less than 5g/100g of saturated fat (A).**
**Foods in (B) are more than 15g/100g of saturated fat,**
**and should be avoided.**
**Foods between 5–15g/100g should be taken in moderation.**

| Food Group | (A) Choose | (B) Avoid eating/drinking |
| --- | --- | --- |
| Cereals | Wholemeal flour<br>Oatmeal<br>Wholegrain bread<br>Wholegrain cereals<br>Porridge<br>Crispbreads<br>Wholegrain rice and pasta | Fancy breads, e.g. croissants, Danish pastries, sponges, choux pastry and all bought cakes, savoury cheese biscuits, cream crackers and biscuits, crisps and savoury snacks |
| Fruit, Vegetables and Salad | All fresh, frozen, dried, bottled or tinned fruit, vegetable and salad, especially peas, beans, lentils, pulses and potatoes (baked or boiled), olives | Chips and roasted potatoes cooked in unsuitable oil or fat (see under Fats) |
| Nuts | Walnuts<br>Almonds<br>Pecan nuts<br>Chestnuts<br>Hazel (filbert) nuts | Coconut |
| Meat | Chicken and turkey (without skin)<br>Veal<br>Lean trimmed grilled steak<br>Rabbit, hare, grouse, partridge, pheasant<br>Venison<br>Soya protein meat substitute | Ham, beef, pork, lamb, bacon, duck, goose offal, liver, kidney, tripe, sweetbreads, heart, brain<br>Crackling and skin<br>Sausages and salami<br>Luncheon meat<br>Pâté, corned beef, Scotch eggs, meat pies and pasties |

| Food group | (A) Choose | (B) Avoid eating/drinking |
|---|---|---|
| Fish | All fresh, frozen, canned, smoked, soused fish<br>Watch tinned fish (olive oil, sunflower oil, brine, tomato sauce permitted, but not vegetable oil) | Battered fish, oily fish and fried fish if you are on a weight reducing diet<br>Fish roe, shellfish: taramásalata, caviar<br>Fish paste (unless made with permitted oils only)<br>Potted fish<br>Fried fish in unsuitable oil or smothered in cheese |
| Eggs and Dairy Produce | Skimmed milk, dried skimmed milk and soya milk. Low fat yoghurt<br>Cottage cheese. Some hard cheeses such as Edam, Brie, Feta and Camembert have lower than average fat content<br>Low fat curd cheese<br>Egg white (meringue) (3 egg yolks per week only) | Whole milk, cream, imitation cream, full fat yoghurt. Ice cream. Evaporated or condensed milk<br>Excess eggs<br>Hard cheese, cream cheese or processed cheese<br>Quiche, soufflé |
| Drinks | Marmite, Bovril, tea, coffee, mineral water, fruit juice | Whole milk drinks, bought soups, cream based liqueurs<br>Malted milk or hot chocolate drinks |
| Sweets, Preserves, Jams and Spreads | Chutney and pickles<br>Sugar-free artificial sweeteners, jam, marmalade, honey | Chocolates, chocolate spreads and sweets. Toffees, fudge, butterscotch, lemon curd |
| Fats | Eat in moderation unsaturated fats, ie. corn oil, sunflower oil, safflower oil, soya oil, olive oil, rapeseed oil, wheatgerm oil, sesame seed oil, poppyseed oil, grapeseed oil<br>Margarine labelled 'high in polyunsaturates' or 'high in linoleic acid' | Saturated fats i.e. butter, dripping, suet, lard, margarine, shortening, ghee, cocoa butter, cooking oil, or vegetable oil of unspecified origin<br>Palm oil, coconut oil, cotton seed oil, peanut oil<br>Peanut butter (especially if hydrogenated) |

# Appendix 3
# Eating out

Going to a restaurant with a partner or friends is something most of us enjoy from time to time, but if you are on a cholesterol-lowering or weight-reducing diet, it can be a disaster! Nowadays Italian, Greek, Turkish, Spanish and Chinese restaurants have tended to anglicise their menus, so that the original cuisine, which should be ideal, is often modified to contain larger amounts of fat than the original version. Indian restaurants probably provide the highest fat cuisine. So, if you do a lot of eating out, sticking to any semblance of a low-fat diet could be a problem. If you are to remain reasonably sociable and don't want to be labelled a food freak, you will have to compromise with your diet on some occasions. But the exception must not become the rule.

The key is to make sure that your diet at home is right and then, when you do eat out, get smart at choosing the best items from the menu. Each kind of ethnic cuisine has its own benefits and potential drawbacks, so here are some tips for healthier food choices from a variety of different menus.

## Chinese

Chinese food tends to be high in complex carbohydrates and low in fat. Stir-fried vegetables, cooked very quickly in a lightly oiled, very hot wok, also retain vitamins better than vegetables cooked in the more traditional way (boiled to death). Chinese restaurants in the UK tend to use more

| Instead of . . . | try |
| --- | --- |
| Egg drop soup | Wonton or hot-and sour soup |
| Egg rolls or fried wontons | Steamed dumplings |
| Fried starters | Boiled, grilled, steamed or very lightly stir-fried starters |
| Dishes with fried meats | Dishes with lots of vegetables |
| Dishes with cashews and peanuts | Dishes with water chestnuts |
| Fried rice | Steamed rice |
| Lobster, black bean, oyster and soy sauce | Sweet and sour sauce, plum or duck sauce |

meat and sauces than those in China, so ask the chef to use only a little oil when preparing your stir-fry and to leave out the soy sauce and monosodium glutamate (very high in salt). Choose dishes with lots of vegetables, such as Chop Suey with steamed rice. Substitute chicken for duck when possible and pass on the crispy fried noodles.

## French

Most people associate French cuisine with rich, salty, heavy sauces, but 'nouvelle cuisine' represents a lighter version. Try to bypass rich starters (e.g. pâté), desserts and sauces, and aim instead for simple dishes, with salads and vegetables.

| Instead of. . . | try |
| --- | --- |
| Starters with olives, capers or anchovies | Less salty options such as steamed mussels or salad |
| Pâté | Steamed mussels |
| French onion soup | Mixed green salad with vinaigrette dressing |
| Croissants | Crusty French bread |
| Hollandaise, Mornay, Béchamel or Béarnaise sauce | Bordelaise or other wine-based sauce |
| Creamy 'au gratin' potato dishes | Lightly sautéed, crisp vegetables |
| Chocolate mousse | Chocolate fat-free pudding |
| Crème caramel | Peaches in wine |

## Greek and Middle Eastern

Some Greek and Middle Eastern dishes are high in fat (usually from olive oil), but others are not. Ask for dishes to be prepared with less oil and for salad dressing and sauces to be served as side dishes. Most Greek sweets are high in fat and sugar. If you really want one, split it with a friend.

| Instead of. . . | try |
| --- | --- |
| Meat-stuffed starters | Starters with rice or aubergine |
| Fried calamari | Dolmades (rice mixture wrapped in vine leaves) |
| Moussaka (lamb and beef casserole) and other creamy or cheesy starters | Roast lamb; shish kebab; couscous or bulgar wheat with vegetables or chicken. |
| Spanakopita (spinach pie with egg and cheese) | Plaki (fish cooked in tomatoes, onions and garlic) |
| Pastries like baklava | Fruit |

## Indian

This cuisine is rich in vegetables, legumes and yogurt. But many Indian dishes are soaked in ghee (clarified butter) or coconut oil, one of the few vegetable oils that consists almost entirely of saturated fatty acids (86 per cent). It's best to start with salads or yogurt topped with chopped or shredded vegetables. Choose chicken or seafood rather than beef or lamb and ask for dishes prepared without ghee.

| Instead of. . . | try |
| --- | --- |
| Samosas (stuffed and fried vegetable pasty) | Papadum or papad (crispy, thin lentil wafers) |
| Korma (braised meat with a rich yogurt cream sauce) | Chicken tikka (roasted in an oven with mild spices) or chicken tandoori (marinated in spices and baked in a clay oven) |
| Curries made with coconut milk or cream | Curries with a vegetable or dal base or tandoori chicken or fish |
| Pakora (deep-fried dough with vegetables) | Gobhi matar tamatar (cauliflower with peas and tomatoes) |
| Saag paneer (spinach with cheese cubes and cream sauce) | Matar pulao (rice pilaf with peas) |
| Sauced rice dishes | Fragrant, steamed rice |
| Fried or stuffed breads | Chapati (thin, dry, whole-wheat bread) or naan (leavened baked bread topped with poppy seeds) |

## Italian

This cuisine – at least the Southern Italian version – is regarded as one of the healthiest in the world (see the Mediterranean Diet – p.221). It's based around pasta, vegetables, fruit and fish. However, the dishes of Northern

| Instead of. . . | try |
| --- | --- |
| Fried calamari | Roasted peppers or minestrone soup |
| Cheese or meat-filled pastas, casserole-type dishes (such as Alfredo sauce) | Pasta primavera (with sautéed garden vegetables) or pasta with white or red clam sauce |
| Pasta with butter or cream sauces | Pasta with Marsala sauce (made with wine) or Marinara sauce (made with tomatoes, onions and garlic) |
| Any scallopine or parmagiana (floured, fried and baked with cheese) dish | Marsala and piccatta cheeses |
| Italian pastries such as cream cake | Italian ices |

Italy are much richer, with a greater use of beef, veal, butter and cream, and studies have shown that residents of northern cities suffer considerably more heart disease than those in the south. Ask the waiter to hold off on the Parmesan cheese, olives and pine nuts and, if you order pizza, choose healthy toppings like spinach, mushrooms, broccoli and roasted peppers.

## Japanese

If anyone has perfected low-fat cuisine, it must be the Japanese, which probably helps to explain the low rates of heart disease in that country. Japanese food highlights rice and vegetables and relies on methods of food preparation that require little or no fat or oil. Unfortunately, however, the traditional Japanese diet is high in salted, smoked or pickled foods, which may be linked to higher rates of stomach cancer and stroke in Japan. Ask the chef to prepare your food without high-sodium marinades, sauces and salt. Ask for any sauces to be served on the side and avoid foods which are deep-fried, battered, breaded or fried.

| Instead of. . . | try |
| --- | --- |
| Vegetable tempura | Steamed vegetables |
| Shrimp tempura | Grilled shrimp or vegetable sushi |
| Tonkatsu (breaded pork cutlet) | Nabemono (casseroles) or Yosenabe (seafood and vegetables in broth) |
| Shabu-Shabu (sliced beef and noodles cooked and served at the table with dipping sauce) | Sukiyaki (beef and vegetables cooked in sauce) or Su udon (hot noodles and broth) |
| Chawan mushi (chicken and shrimp in egg custard) | Chicken or beef teriyaki (grilled) |

*Note:* **Above based on recommendations of the American Heart Association.**

# Appendix 4
# Sample activity programmes

## A SIMPLE STRETCHING EXERCISES

Before – and immediately after – you walk, jog or cycle, it's a good idea to do some gentle stretching exercises. Remember not to bounce when you stretch. Perform the movements slowly and stretch as far as you feel comfortable.

### Side reaches

Reach one arm over your head and to the side. Keep your hips steady and your shoulders straight to the side. Hold for 10 seconds and repeat on the other side.

### Wall push

Place your hands on a wall with your feet about three to four feet away from the wall. Keep your back leg straight with your foot flat and your toes pointed straight ahead. Lean forward gently, until you feel the calf muscle in the rear leg begin to stretch. Hold for 10 seconds and repeat with the other leg to the rear.

### Knee pull

Lean your back against a wall. Keep your head, hips, and feet in a straight line. Pull one knee to your chest, hold for 10 seconds, then repeat with the other leg.

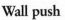

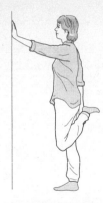

**Leg curl**
Pull your foot to your buttocks with your opposite hand. Keep your knee pointing straight to the ground. Hold for 10 seconds and repeat with the other hand.

## B  WALKING

When you begin walking, make sure you:
- Walk with your chin up and your shoulders held slightly back.
- Wear suitable footwear, with good ankle support.
- Walk so that the heel of your foot touches the ground first and roll your weight forward.
- Walk with your toes pointed forward and swing your arms as you walk.

If you are recovering from a heart attack or heart surgery, complete the eight-week preliminary walking programme (p.147) before starting on the schedule below.

*Note:* **You should aim to walk on four or five occasions per week.**

| | Warm up time | Fast Walk time | Cool Down time | Total time |
|---|---|---|---|---|
| Week 1 | Walk slowly 5 min. | Walk briskly 5 min. | Walk slowly 5 min. | 15 min. |
| Week 2 | Walk slowly 5 min. | Walk briskly 7 min. | Walk slowly 5 min. | 17 min. |
| Week 3 | Walk slowly 5 min. | Walk briskly 9 min. | Walk slowly 5 min. | 19 min. |
| Week 4 | Walk slowly 5 min. | Walk briskly 11 min. | Walk slowly 5 min. | 21 min. |
| Week 5 | Walk slowly 5 min. | Walk briskly 13 min. | Walk slowly 5 min. | 23 min. |
| Week 6 | Walk slowly 5 min. | Walk briskly 15 min. | Walk slowly 5 min. | 25 min |
| Week 7 | Walk slowly 5 min. | Walk briskly 18 min. | Walk slowly 5 min. | 28 min. |
| Week 8 | Walk slowly 5 min. | Walk briskly 20 min. | Walk slowly 5 min. | 30 min. |
| Week 9 | Walk slowly 5 min. | Walk briskly 23 min. | Walk slowly 5 min. | 33 min. |
| Week 10 | Walk slowly 5 min. | Walk briskly 26 min. | Walk slowly 5 min. | 36 min. |
| Week 11 | Walk slowly 5 min. | Walk briskly 28 min. | Walk slowly 5 min. | 38 min. |
| Week 12 | Walk slowly 5 min. | Walk briskly 30 min. | Walk slowly 5 min. | 40 min. |

For **Week 13** and beyond, gradually increase your brisk walking time to 30–60 minutes four or five times a week.

# C  JOGGING

If you are over the age of 40 and have not been active, you should not begin with a programme as strenuous as jogging. Start with the walking programme instead. After completing the 12-week walking programme, you can start at week 3 of the jogging programme. Note that:

- You should aim to jog on four or five occasions per week.
- Each session consists of walking for five minutes, followed by some stretching exercises, followed by walking/jogging and ending with a three minute walk and a further two minute stretch.
- Stretching exercises can be found at the beginning of this section.

| | Warm up | Jogging phase | Cool down | Total time |
|---|---|---|---|---|
| Week 1 | Walk 5 min. then stretch | Walk briskly for 10 min. | Walk 3 min. stretch 2 min. | 20 min. |
| Week 2 | Walk 5 min. then stretch | Walk 5 min, jog 1 min. walk 5 min, jog 1 min. | Walk 3 min. stretch 2 min. | 22 min. |
| Week 3 | Walk 5 min. then stretch | Walk 5 min, jog 3 min. walk 5 min, jog 3 min. | Walk 3 min. stretch 2 min. | 26 min. |
| Week 4 | Walk 5 min. then stretch | Walk 4 min, jog 5 min. walk 4 min, jog 5 min. | Walk 3 min. stretch 2 min. | 28 min. |
| Week 5 | Walk 5 min. then stretch | Walk 4 min, jog 5 min. walk 4 min, jog 5 min. | Walk 3 min. stretch 2 min. | 28 min. |
| Week 6 | Walk 5 min. then stretch | Walk 4 min, jog 6 min. walk 4 min, jog 6 min. | Walk 3 min. stretch 2 min. | 30 min. |
| Week 7 | Walk 5 min. then stretch | Walk 4 min, jog 7 min. walk 4 min, jog 7 min. | Walk 3 min. stretch 2 min. | 32 min. |
| Week 8 | Walk 5 min. then stretch | Walk 4 min, jog 8 min. walk 4 min, jog 8 min. | Walk 3 min. stretch 2 min. | 34 min. |
| Week 9 | Walk 5 min. then stretch | Walk 4 min, jog 9 min. walk 4 min, jog 9 min. | Walk 3 min. stretch 2 min. | 36 min. |
| Week 10 | Walk 5 min. then stretch | Walk 4 min. jog 13 min. | Walk 3 min. stretch 2 min. | 27 min. |
| Week 11 | Walk 5 min. then stretch | Walk 4 min. jog 15 min. | Walk 3 min. stretch 2 min. | 29 min. |
| Week 12 | Walk 5 min. then stretch | Walk 4 min. jog 17 min. | Walk 3 min. stretch 2 min. | 31 min. |
| Week 13 | Walk 5 min. then stretch | Walk 2 min. jog 19 min. | Walk 3 min. stretch 2 min. | 31 min. |
| Week 14 | Walk 5 min. then stretch | Walk 1 min. jog 20 min. | Walk 3 min. stretch 2 min. | 31 min. |
| Week 15 | Walk 5 min. then stretch | Jog 20 min. | Walk 3 min. stretch 2 min. | 30 min. |

For **Week 16** and beyond, aim to jog for 30 minutes on four or five occasions per week.

## D  CYCLING

The cycling programmes have been designed for cycling on an ordinary touring or mountain bicycle. The choice of gears has no influence on the programme. You should:

- Use the build-up programme for your age category.
- When you have completed level 10 of the build-up programme, you can move on to the maintenance programme.
- Always wear a crash helmet.

Build-up programme for age range 30–39 years

| Stage | Distance (km) | (miles) | Time (minutes) | Speed (km/hr) | (mph) | Number of times per week |
|-------|------|--------|--------|--------|-------|--------|
| 1 | 7·5 | 4·7 | 30 | 15·0 | 9·3 | 5 |
| 2 | 8·0 | 5·0 | 30 | 16·0 | 9·9 | 5 |
| 3 | 9·0 | 5·6 | 30 | 18·0 | 11·2 | 4 |
| 4 | 10·5 | 6·5 | 35 | 18·0 | 11·2 | 4 |
| 5 | 11·0 | 6·8 | 35 | 18·8 | 11·7 | 4 |
| 6 | 12·5 | 7·8 | 40 | 18·8 | 11·7 | 4 |
| 7 | 14·0 | 8·7 | 45 | 18·7 | 11·6 | 4 |
| 8 | 15·0 | 9·3 | 45 | 20·0 | 12·4 | 4 |
| 9 | 15·5 | 9·6 | 45 | 20·6 | 12·8 | 4 |
| 10 | 16·0 or 16·0 | 9·9 or 9·9 | 45 50 | 21·3 19·2 | 13·2 11·9 | 4 4 |

Then continue with the maintenance programme.

Build-up programme for age range 40–49 years

| Stage | Distance (km) | (miles) | Time (minutes) | Speed (km/hr) | (mph) | Number of times per week |
|-------|------|--------|--------|--------|-------|--------|
| 1 | 6·0 | 3·7 | 25 | 14·4 | 8·9 | 5 |
| 2 | 7·5 | 4·7 | 30 | 15·0 | 9·3 | 5 |
| 3 | 10·0 | 6·2 | 40 | 15·0 | 9·3 | 4 |
| 4 | 11·5 | 7·1 | 40 | 17·2 | 10·7 | 4 |
| 5 | 12·5 | 7·8 | 40 | 18·8 | 11·7 | 4 |
| 6 | 13·0 | 8·1 | 40 | 19·5 | 12·1 | 4 |
| 7 | 15·0 | 9·3 | 50 | 18·0 | 11·2 | 4 |
| 8 | 15·0 | 9·3 | 45 | 20·0 | 12·4 | 4 |
| 9 | 16·0 | 9·9 | 50 | 19·2 | 11·9 | 4 |
| 10 | 16·0 or 16·0 | 9·9 or 9·9 | 45 50 | 21·3 19·2 | 13·2 11·9 | 4 4 |

Then continue with the maintenance programme.

Build-up programme for age 50 years and over

| Stage | Distance (km) | (miles) | Time (minutes) | Speed (km/hr) | (mph) | Number of times per week |
|---|---|---|---|---|---|---|
| 1 | 6·0 or | 3·7 or | 30 or | 12·0 or | 7·5 or | 5 |
|   | 6·0 | 3·7 | 25 | 14·4 | 8·9 | |
| 2 | 7·5 | 4·7 | 30 | 15·0 | 9·3 | 5 |
| 3 | 9·0 | 5·6 | 35 | 15·4 | 9·6 | 4 |
| 4 | 10·5 | 6·5 | 40 | 15·8 | 9·8 | 4 |
| 5 | 12·5 | 7·8 | 50 | 15·0 | 9·3 | 4 |
| 6 | 12·5 | 7·8 | 45 | 16·7 | 10·4 | 4 |
| 7 | 14·0 | 8·7 | 50 | 16·8 | 10·4 | 4 |
| 8 | 14·0 | 8·7 | 45 | 18·7 | 11·6 | 4 |
| 9 | 16·0 | 9·9 | 55 | 17·5 | 10·9 | 4 |
| 10 | 16·0 or | 9·9 or | 50 | 19·2 | 11·9 | 4 |
|   | 18·0 or | 11·2 or | 60 | 18·0 | 11·2 | 4 |
|   | 16·0 | 9·9 | 55 | 17·5 | 10·9 | 5 |

Then continue with the maintenance programme.

Maintenance cycling programme for all ages

| Distance (km) | (miles) | Time (minutes) | Speed (km/hr) | (mph) | Number of times per week |
|---|---|---|---|---|---|
| 10·0 or | 6·2 or | 25 | 24·0 | 14·9 | 6 |
| 12·0 or | 7·5 or | 35 | 20·6 | 12·8 | 6 |
| 13·0 or | 8·1 or | 35 | 22·0 | 13·7 | 5 |
| 14·0 or | 8·7 or | 45 | 18·7 | 11·6 | 5 |
| 16·0 or | 9·9 or | 45 | 21·3 | 13·2 | 4 |
| 17·0 or | 10·6 or | 55 | 18·5 | 11·4 | 4 |
| 17·5 or | 10·9 or | 45 | 23·3 | 14·5 | 3 |
| 20·0 | 12·4 | 60 | 20·0 | 12·4 | 3 |

# Abbreviations

| | |
|---|---|
| ACE | angiotensin converting enzyme |
| APMHR | age predicted maximum heart rate |
| BP | blood pressure |
| CABG | coronary artery bypass graft |
| CAT | computerised axial tomography |
| CHD | coronary heart disease |
| CRP | C-reactive protein |
| CVD | cardiovascular disease |
| DASH | Dietary Approaches to Stop Hypertension |
| DBP | diastolic blood pressure |
| DNA | deoxyribonucleic acid |
| DVLA | Driver and Vehicle Licensing Agency |
| ECG | electrocardiogram – resting and exercise |
| GI | Glycaemic Index |
| GTN | glyceryl trinitrate |
| HDL-C | high-density lipoprotein cholesterol |
| HERS | Heart and Oestrogen/Progestogen Replacement Study |
| HRT | hormone replacement therapy |
| ISH | isolated systolic hypertension |
| IU | international unit |
| LDL-C | low-density lipoprotein cholesterol |
| MCA | Medicines Control Agency |
| mg/100ml | milligrams per 100 millilitres |
| mmHG | millimetres of mercury |
| mmol/L | millimoles per litre |
| MRI | magnetic resonance imaging |
| NIDDM | non-insulin dependent diabetes |
| OC | oral contraceptive |
| PET | positron emission tomography |
| PCOS | polycystic ovarian syndrome |
| PUFA | polyunsaturated fat |
| RDA | recommended daily allowances |
| RMR | resting metabolic rate |
| SBP | systolic blood pressure |
| TC | total cholesterol |
| TMLR | transmyocardial laser revascularisation |

# Glossary

**ACE inhibitor**  A drug. ACE stands for angiotensin converting enzyme.

**Aerobic exercise**  Regular, rhythmic exercise involving major muscle groups which improve the functioning of the heart and circulation. Examples include brisk walking, swimming and cycling.

**Aneurysm**  A balloon like swelling in an artery, or in the heart.

**Angina (angina pectoris)**  Pain, heaviness or tightness in the chest which may spread to the neck, jaw or arms. Occurs when the coronary arteries have become so narrow that insufficient oxygen-rich blood can reach the heart muscle when demands are high, such as during physical exertion.

**Angiography**  A special X-ray of the arteries. See Coronary Angiography.

**Angioplasty**  A treatment which improves the blood flow through an artery. See Coronary Angioplasty.

**Anti-arrhythmic drug**  A drug used to control a disorder of heart rhythm.

**Anti-platelet drugs**  A drug used to thin the blood and prevent clotting, by reducing the 'stickiness' of platelets – the tiny blood cells that clump together to help form a clot.

**Anticoagulant**  Also used to prevent blood clots. Clots consist of two elements: platelets which clump together and a protein called *fibrin*. Anticoagulants act by preventing formation of fibrin.

**Antioxidants**  Vitamins E, C and beta-carotene, found in fresh fruit and vegetables. May help to reduce the build-up of fatty plaque (atheroma) in the arterial wall.

**Aorta**  The main blood vessel of the heart.

**Arrhythmia**  A disorder of the heart rhythm.

**Artery**  Muscular-walled tubes which carry oxygen-enriched blood from the heart to the tissues and organs of the body.

**Aspirin**  An anti-platelet drug used to reduce the risk of blood clots.

**Atheroma**  The name given to the fatty material that can build up in the walls of the arteries. When it affects the coronary arteries it can cause angina or heart attack. When it involves the arteries of the brain, a stroke may result. See also Plaque.

**Atherosclerosis**  The *process* by which fatty material builds up in the arteries.

**Atrial fibrillation**  A common disorder of heart rhythm which may cause breathlessness, heart failure or blood clots.

**Beta-blockers**  These drugs block the action of adrenaline on the heart and blood vessels thus slowing the heart and making it beat less forcefully. Used to treat angina and hypertension.

**Bile resins** Drugs used to lower cholesterol levels. Cholestyramine and colestipol are examples.

**Blood cholesterol** See Cholesterol.

**Blood lipids** The collective term for all the fatty substances in the blood including LDL-Cholesterol, HDL-Cholesterol and triglycerides.

**Blood pressure** The pressure of the blood in the arteries. The highest pressure (known as the systolic pressure) occurs when the heart contracts and forces blood through the system. The lowest pressure (diastolic pressure) occurs when the heart rests between beats. Blood pressure is measured in millimetres of mercury (mmHg), eg. 120/70 mmHg.

**Body Mass Index (BMI)** A measure of weight relative to height used to determine whether someone is overweight. Calculated as follows: BMI=Weight (kg)/ Height (Metres $^2$). Those with a BMI over 30 Kg/m $^2$ are considered obese.

**Calcium antagonists** Class of drugs used to treat angina and hypertension. Also called calcium channel blockers.

**Cardiac** To do with the heart.

**Cardiac Rehabilitation** A structured programme for people who have had a heart attack or heart surgery, consisting of exercise, relaxation and information on lifestyle and treatment.

**Cardiovascular Disease (CVD)** A collective term including coronary heart disease, stroke and all other diseases of the heart and circulation.

**Cholesterol** It is a soft waxy substance found in all the cells of the body, especially those of the brain, spinal cord and nerves. Cholesterol is carried in the bloodstream by special proteins called lipoproteins. High levels of blood cholesterol are associated with increased risk of heart disease.

**Clot-buster** Special drugs used in the acute phase of a heart attack to dissolve blood clot in the blocked coronary artery. See also Thrombolytics.

**Coronary Angiography** A special X-ray of the coronary arteries. A fine tube called a catheter is introduced into the artery in the arm or groin and passed through to where the coronary arteries originate. A special dye is then injected which can be seen on X-ray and which produces a 'road map' of the arteries, showing where the arteries are narrowed and the severity of the narrowing.

**Coronary Angioplasty** A treatment which improves blood flow through the coronary arteries. A fine catheter (hollow tube) with a small inflatable balloon at the tip, is inserted into the coronary arteries and passed through to the areas where the narrowing is most severe. The balloon is then inflated and crushes the fatty plaque into the arterial wall, thus opening the artery and improving blood flow.

**Coronary Artery Bypass Grafting (CABG)** Major heart surgery requiring a hospital stay of some five to seven days. Diseased arteries are bypassed by grafting a blood vessel between the aorta and a point in the coronary artery beyond the narrowed or blocked area. A single, two, three or four grafts may be required.

**Coronary Heart Disease (CHD)** When the walls of the coronary arteries become narrowed by the gradual build-up of plaque or atheroma. Typical symptoms of CHD include breathlessness and angina, or a heart attack. Also known as ischaemic heart disease.

**Coronary thrombosis** Also known as a heart attack or myocardial infarction.

**Digitalis (digoxin)** A drug used in the treatment of heart failure and certain disorders of heart rhythm. It is made from the foxglove plant, digitalis.

**Diuretics** Also called water tablets. They increase the amount of salt and water passed in the urine and are used to treat high blood pressure and heart failure.

**Echocardiography** An investigation which uses sound beams to take pictures of the heart (the same instrument which takes pictures of a baby in the womb). With this type of scanner it is possible to see the heart muscle contracting and to identify areas that are contracting poorly because of poor blood supply from the coronary arteries.

**Electrocardiogram (ECG)** A test to record the rhythm and activity of the heart. It can be used at rest or when the patient is exercising on a treadmill – an exercise electrocardiogram.

**Familial Hyperlipidaemia (FH)** An inherited condition in which the blood cholesterol is very high.

**Fibrates** A class of drugs which reduce triglycerides, increase HDL-cholesterol and lower total cholesterol with the net effect of lowering coronary risk. Bezafibrate and Gemfibrozil are examples.

**Fibrinogen** A blood protein involved in the clotting process. High levels are associated with an increased risk of heart disease.

**Glycaemic Index (GI)** A measures of how fast the carbohydrate of a particular food is converted to glucose and enters the blood stream.

**Glyceryl Trinitrate (GTN)** Also called nitroglycerin. A highly effective drug for the relief of angina.

**Heart Attack** See Myocardial infarction.

**Heart Failure** When the pumping action of the heart is inadequate to fulfil the demands of the body for blood. Nowadays, heart failure can be controlled with modern drugs.

**High-density lipoprotein cholesterol (HDL-C)** Often known as the 'good cholesterol', HDL-C helps to protect the heart by returning excess cholesterol from the arteries to the liver.

**Homocysteine** A product of dietary protein. Elevated blood levels of homocysteine are associated with an increased risk of cardiovascular disease.

**Hormone Replacement Therapy (HRT)** A combination of oestrogen and progestogen used to treat menopausal symptoms and to prevent osteoporosis. It is not yet clear whether HRT protects against heart disease.

**Hydrogenation** A process whereby hydrogen is added to unsaturated fats so that they become firmer at room temperature. Manufacturers use it to prolong shelf-life and improve food texture.

**Hypercholesterolaemia** Raised blood cholesterol.

**Hypertension** High blood pressure.

**Insulin Resistance Syndrome (IRS)** A condition in which abdominal (central) fat leads to high blood pressure, abnormal blood lipids and diabetes, all of which increase the risk of heart disease.

**Ischaemia** When the coronary arteries are narrowed and unable to allow sufficient blood to reach the heart muscle.

**Isometric exercise** Exercises in which muscle tension is produced without moving a joint e.g. lifting heavy weights.

**Lipoproteins** Special carriers by means of which cholesterol and other lipids – which cannot dissolve in the blood – are transported to and from the cells.

**Low density lipoprotein cholesterol (LDL-C)** Also known as the 'bad cholesterol'. The main form of cholesterol in the blood, high levels of LDL-C are associated with an increased risk of heart attack.

**Magnetic Resonance Imaging (MRI)** A diagnostic tool that uses a magnetic field rather than X-rays or sound waves to create three-dimensional images of internal organs.

**Monounsaturated fat** A type of fat found in olive oil, sunflower oil, rapeseed oil and in some margarines and spreads. Monounsaturated fats have a single double bond in their carbon chain. They may help to lower blood levels of LDL-C – the harmful form of cholesterol.

**Morbidity Rate** The proportion of people in the community who have symptoms of heart or circulatory disease such as angina, heart failure or hypertension.

**Mortality Rate** The number of deaths from heart or circulatory disease.

**Myocardial infarction** The medical term for a heart attack. Occurs when one of the three coronary arteries is blocked by a blood clot (thrombosis), starving a portion of the heart muscle of oxygen-rich blood.

**Myocardium** The medical term for heart muscle.

**Nitrates** The most commonly used class of drugs for the treatment of angina. They relax the muscle layer in the walls of the coronary arteries making them wider and thus improving blood flow to the heart.

**Non-insulin Dependent Diabetes Mellitus (NIDDM)** Also known as 'maturity onset' or 'Type II' diabetes. Usually occurs over the age of 40 and is commonly associated with obesity.

**Obesity** An excess of fat cells. Obesity is associated with an increased risk of cardiovascular disease.

**Oestrogen** Along with progestogen, one of the main female sex hormones. Increases HDL-C whilst lowering LDL-C, thus reducing the risk of heart disease.

**Osteoporosis** A condition of brittle and fragile bones caused by loss of bone mineral, especially as a result of hormonal changes, or deficiency of calcium or vitamin D.

**Plaque**  Fatty deposits in the arteries (also known as atheroma).

**Polyunsaturated fats (PUFAs)**  Polyunsaturated fats tend to have a liquid consistency whether at room or refrigerator temperature and have two or more double bonds in their carbon chain structure. There are two families of PUFA in the diet: the Omega 6 (derived from linoleic acid) and the Omega 3 (derived from alpha linoleic acid). Eating these fats rather than saturated fats may help to lower blood cholesterol levels.

**Potassium channel activators**  New drugs, which act in a similar way to nitrates, causing relaxation of the coronary arteries and hence improved blood flow.

**Progestogen**  Along with oestrogen, one of the main female sex hormones. Tends to work in the opposite way to oestrogen by increasing LDL-C and reducing HDL-C thus tending to increase the risk of heart disease.

**Resting Metabolic Rate (RMR)**  The energy we use at rest just to maintain normal body functions such as breathing, digestion etc. It accounts for about 60 per cent of our daily energy expenditure.

**Saturated fat**  A type of fat found mainly in food from animal sources, particularly dairy foods and meat products. Saturated fats have no double bonds in their carbon chain structure and tend to be solid at room temperature. Diets rich in saturated fat increase blood cholesterol levels and the risk of heart disease.

**Statins**  A highly effective group of drugs used to lower blood cholesterol levels. Examples include Simvastatin and Pravastatin.

**Stent**  A short tube of stainless steel mesh, inserted into the coronary artery at the section of the artery to be widened during angioplasty. The stent is left in place to prevent further arterial narrowing at this point.

**Stroke**  Damage to the brain resulting from a blood clot blocking the arteries supplying blood to the brain, or from a haemorrhage into the brain substance.

**Syndrome X**  Also known as variant angina. A variety of chest pain which mimics typical cardiac pain but in which the coronary arteries are normal. More common in women.

**Thrombolytics**  Clot busting drugs which can stop a heart attack by dissolving the clot if given within the first few hours.

**Thrombosis**  Medical term for a blood clot.

**Total cholesterol**  Refers to the total amount of cholesterol in the blood, i.e. the sum of LDL-Cholesterol, HDL-Cholesterol and the small amounts contained in other lipoproteins.

**Trans fats**  These are a special group of fats which are produced during the commercial process of hydrogenation. Trans fats increase cholesterol levels and may, therefore, increase the risk of heart disease.

**Transmyocardial Laser Revascularisation (TMLR)**  A new procedure still being researched whereby a small incision is made in the chest wall and a powerful laser is used to 'drill' 30–40 holes through the heart muscle itself. This enables oxygen-rich blood to reach areas of the heart muscle previously starved of blood because of narrowed arteries.

**Triglycerides** A form of blood lipid (fat), high levels of which appear to increase the risk of heart disease in women but not in men. They are fats that come from our diet or are manufactured by the body.

**Unsaturated fat** A type of fat which has one or more double bond in the carbon chain and which tends to be liquid at room temperature. There are two groups of unsaturated fats depending upon how many double bonds are in the carbon chain i.e. monounsaturated (one double bond) or polyunsaturated (two or more double bonds).

**Venous thrombosis** Blood clots in the deep veins of the legs.

# Index